GW01044109

Memories of a Mental Nurse

By

Robert Panton

Also by this author:

‘ Holy Roller.’

and ‘Memories of an Alzheimers Night Nurse.’

Introduction.

"They're different, not quite the run of the mill.

People with a mental illness, particularly those suffering from a psychosis aren't quite 'the thing' are they? You might smile at them, or sometimes one could feel afraid of them, because they aren't the norm and not generally the type of people you'd look on as close friends.

Before I became a psychiatric nurse I, probably like most other people in the mid seventies, knew there were unfortunate individuals who lived up in the big building just outside of town, surrounded by a high wall and metal railings, and the people who lived there weren't really part of our society.

These people existed in a world of their own and were certainly not the type that you were likely to come across in everyday life, not the sort that you needed to bother about.

As a lad if I misbehaved, my mum would tell me in a rather menacing manner obviously meaning to frighten me.

"If you don't watch yourself boy, the man in the green van will take you away to the asylum where all the funny people go."

This was often the threat, unless I conformed to what she thought of as 'normal behaviour.'

No, these weren't people that I intended to get involved with!

Later on as a psychiatric nurse I realised that those who suffered with mental health problems were people in their own right, just like the ordinary man or woman in the street and they had feelings just as I had, and their feelings were often muddled due to the illnesses that they sadly lived with.

In fact I soon came to realise that they were all different, not just a bunch of odd unfortunates, shut away in a big mental hospital locked up out of the way of normal people, but each one of them had their own personalities, their own concerns, their own worries and cares and often their own interests, just like the local shopkeeper, the deliveryman, or the factory worker. Despite their various illnesses they were real men and women who had differing personalities like everyone else. Most of the patients I was about to meet in my chosen career were as about 'normal' as you and I in their earlier lives, but the trauma and the stigma of mental illness changed everything for them, whether it was a psychotic illness, or a breakdown due to a bereavement, or stress; often life would never be the same for them again.

In the seventies when I began my nurse training most people suffering with a severe mental illness or breakdown, often ended up at least for a time in one of the many large mental hospitals which were usually situated on the edge of our towns and cities.

"Best to keep them separate from normal people," was the old thinking.

Nowadays of course, things are different most of those institutions have been closed down and have either been turned into museums, or have been demolished to make way for housing estates.

A lot of the care for people suffering with a mental illness is now undertaken in the community, but the stigma is still there, though hopefully at a much lower level, as communities get used to seeing people with mental illnesses living among them. Some of the old hospitals continue to function, but are much smaller in size and a lot of their activity is with outpatients, or they provide 'drop in' facilities for people needing support away from a ward environment.

I'd like to tell you of my experiences of nursing in those earlier days and to show that, despite the reputation the old psychiatric hospitals had among the general population, they were actually a haven to many and in fact, when they were closed many patients didn't want to leave. Due to the length of time they had spent there they looked upon the hospital as their home, with the staff and the other patients as part of their family. Some, probably many, throughout the country actually committed suicide rather than leave what had been home, for the majority of their lives. This is merely pointing out that though there may be a lot of good things about the present system of caring for mentally ill people in the community there was, I firmly believe a lot of good in the old system as well.

To some, the things I write about may sometimes seem repugnant, but I can only tell it as I remember it. To others it might seem that there's a lot political incorrectness, even in the extreme, but what must be remembered is that the beginning of my recollection was almost forty years ago.

There wasn't a Health and Safety act as far as I am aware, and even if in the unlikely event there was, it would have been a beast without teeth. Political correctness was yet to be invented, you could treat minority groups just as you liked within reason and indeed there were many injustices in society and a great deal of suspicion of 'foreigners,' not though, strangely enough in nursing; not at least in psychiatric nursing, which was a blessing as I rather liked some of the people from the many different nations that I worked with.

Sadly in those days Psychiatric nurses were looked upon by many general nurses as little more than ‘attendants,’ with no real knowledge of the illnesses that were dealt with in a general hospital, at least that’s how a lot of us in mental health nursing felt, but psychiatric training included much that was in general nurse training, though of course there were differences, but to have seen us as uneducated was unfair, especially as we performed a lot of the clinical procedures that would have been undertaken in a general hospital. Perhaps, if indeed we were looked upon as second-class nurses it was maybe our own attitude, as so often when in the presence of a general nurse, we referred to her as a ‘real’ nurse.

The names of staff and patients have been changed, even my own, for what I hope are obvious reasons and sometimes I may have some of the facts slightly out of order or occasionally incorrect, after all much of it was a long time ago and my mind is not as young and as agile as it was. Nevertheless, the account that I have given is reasonably accurate and the events certainly are true events to the best of my memory.

Bear in mind though, that some of the terminology and names of illness have altered over the years, e.g. what is called mental health now, was then known as mental illness; manic depressive illness has for some reason or other, become bi-polar disorder. For anyone who is familiar with modern trends, names and terminology I'll probably sound rather antiquated throughout this account; I hope that I'll be forgiven!

Much of what the following pages contain of course, recounts my own history as well as the hopes and aspirations, the triumphs and the disappointments that I experienced during my years, as a psychiatric nurse and I think that there were many others who may have gone through the same turmoil's and ultimately the same joys and sense of satisfaction that I experienced in this, a most rewarding of occupations.

'Mental nursing' was a peculiar job, quite unlike any other. One moment there would be laughter, another tears, then perhaps anger, or fear, and occasionally (perhaps more than occasionally) despair. All of these emotions would be seen in many of the staff, or experienced in oneself, and perhaps all in the one day.

There was one thing for sure though, things were never dull and one felt that ones life was not only worthwhile, but that it was so very often full of things that made you chuckle, or even caused you to roar with laughter.

Laughter, if it could be shared with the patients, as it often could be, was as good as any medication. I truly hope that there will be many more that will follow in the footsteps of the psychiatric nurse, perhaps even some who read through this book!

It has been a privilege to be in such an occupation and, even if you’ve no knowledge of nursing and no desire to be a nurse I hope that this little history will prove interesting, enlightening and though, sometimes tragic, but often amusing.

Chapter I

Life was quite comfortable for me in 1974; I was twenty-five years old and earning a reasonable wage, driving a van delivering groceries to caterers. My days were quite easy, starting at eight and finishing, if I was lucky at twelve, then whiling away the rest of the day by the side of the nearest river, or sleeping in a lay-by for a couple of hours, so as not to arrive at the depot too early and be forced into doing some of the warehouse work which always awaited those who were foolish enough to return before their time.

It was a good job as far as it went and I certainly couldn't grumble about the wages, but I wasn't happy. Earlier in my working life I had been a bakers rounds-man and all had gone well until the dark day that I had accidentally backed my wagon into a ditch. That might have been excusable on any other day, but this was a seaside resort and the people who were waiting for their bread were owners of cafes and restaurants, or people who ran burger bars and bed and breakfasts. It was the busiest weekend of the year;

an august bank holiday and they lost a fantastic amount of money. They couldn't forgive me and who can blame them?

After that disaster I left the bakery and became the manager of a boutique, but the shop was so far down the high street that customers were very few and far between and I and my assistant became so bored that we started to imitate the customers behind their backs, which was ok until one of them noticed me in the mirror, imitating and mocking him. How I didn't get a bloody nose, or the sack I'll never know!

One day the area manager paid me a visit and noticed that on a particular Wednesday, (which was half day closing and always very quiet,) our takings were nil.

"In all my years in retail trading, I've never known a shop to take nothing," he said in disgust. My fate was sealed!

Nevertheless, looking back I really believe that even if I had been successful in my working life there was something more I needed to do; I was dissatisfied, the days dragged by without any real meaning and I longed to do something that was worthwhile, driving a delivery van was ok. But it didn't satisfy my need to be useful.

One of my problems was that I was an active member of an evangelical church and having done children's work and youth work in the church, I wanted to spread my wings and become a pastor. That wasn't easy in those days, because to go to Bible College and train for the ministry would cost money and I couldn't get a grant. I had a wife and two children to support, so as far as the ministry was concerned there was no possibility of me fulfilling my ambitions in that area. So I was in a bit of a state; I didn't want to do mundane jobs however well paid they were, I wanted to do something that had real meaning.

Fortunately my auntie worked in the local psychiatric hospital. She was in the administration department working as a welfare officer. One particular day while feeling really frustrated with things and unfulfilled in my life, I began to talk to her about my situation.

"I feel like my life is going nowhere," I told her,

"I want something more fulfilling and more of a challenge."

"Well I know they're looking for staff at St. Andrews, I could put a good word in for you with one of the nursing officers at the hospital and try and arrange for you to meet somebody to talk things over with. Perhaps you might be able to do your training, I'm not sure whether you need any 'O' levels, but you can always ask." She said, reassuringly.

Incidentally the hospital she was working at was the very one where my great grandfather had been the chief male attendant in the 1800's when the hospital was known as an Asylum!

Not wanting to jump into something before I had a proper idea of what to expect, I went along to the local job centre and collected what little information they had on psychiatric nursing. One of the leaflets that I came across, encouraging young people especially, to join the psychiatric nursing force, showed on the front cover a photograph of a young man in a white coat sitting alongside his patient on a bench within the hospital grounds. The patient appeared to be pouring out his troubles to the nurse. I pictured myself as that nurse, giving the appropriate advice to the distressed patient and of course releasing him from all of his problems, then sending him on his way a new man, and I myself, quite naturally feeling suitably proud of my achievement. Then in my minds eye in all saintly humility looking around quickly, in order to help as many other poor unfortunates as I could and to allow as many as possible to benefit from my undoubted abilities in this field.

After all it was in the blood, wasn't it? Hadn't my great grandfather risen to dizzy heights in this field of service?

What a worthwhile job!

‘This beats carting boxes of peas and potatoes about,’ I said to myself.

In fact, I thought, with my special aptitude for this type of work I could do a great deal towards reducing the seven hundred, or so beds in the hospital and who knows, perhaps other hospitals would hear of my talents and I could become a sort of consultant, travelling the countryside and bringing relief to thousands of tortured souls, a sort of modern day St. Peter who as he passed by, even his shadow would bring healing to the sick and needy. Poor deluded man that I was, little did I realise at that point how different it was all going to be.

Shortly afterwards my auntie arranged a meeting for me with one of the nursing officers whom I met at the main entrance to the hospital one evening for an informal chat.

I don’t remember much about the meeting, only that it was six o’ clock one summers evening and I was tired, having been out at work all that hot, sticky day. I had gone straight home from work and had a bath, changed my clothes, eaten something hurriedly, then gone straight out afterwards not wanting to be late. Turning my car into the hospital grounds, I slowly made my way up the long drive, which was bordered by beautiful coloured begonia beds and with beautifully kept lush, green lawns sweeping away, on either side.

Parking my old banger in one of the few places available in front of a magnificent Victorian limestone building, I looked up in nervous anticipation. The facade that contained the reception area reminded me of a stately home, every bit as grand and imposing, it was beautiful. At that moment, due to my nervous state I wasn't overly interested, yet I couldn't help but be at least subconsciously impressed because I remembered it well later, and I can still recall it today.

I was trembling and wanted to use the toilet, never having liked interviews even informal ones, and this massive building with all the other large hospital houses around, was awesome and somehow scary; it all seemed to stretch on forever. Besides I thought, what might lie beyond and behind it and what would the person inside, who had arranged to meet me, be like? However, here I was so I'd better get on with it.

'Not the time to chicken out now,' I told myself.

Getting out of the car I walked slowly towards the great wooden doors that stood open, revealing a large imposing reception area, tastefully decorated.

"Mr. Panton?"

A short stocky man who spoke with an Irish accent and who looked to me typically Irish, (if that is possible) approached me and held out his hand, which I shook briefly as we introduced ourselves.

This was Paddy O'Rourke not at all like of some of the other nursing officers I would come across later. He seemed a kindly, homely sort of man, not threatening, unlike many I met while doing my training, and later on as a staff nurse. For all that he was a kind man though, to me he was always Mr. O'Rourke, never Paddy, however friendly he might have been; apart from the fact that I had always been in awe of authority and would never have dared to have been on first name terms with a superior. I learned that nursing officers were usually called Mr. or, Miss. so and so, never, except by a few privileged few, by their first name's. All of that seems to have gone by the board nowadays of course, with even many of the doctors known by their Christian or, first names, I blame it all on the TV soaps!

Following our introduction, Mr. O'Rourke said with his lovely Irish lilt,

"If you come down to the nursing office with me, we'll have a little chat about things. Your aunt seems quite keen to get you started and speaks highly of you."

“Thank you,” I murmured nervously, hardly able to get my mouth to speak any words.

It’s a strange thing anxiety, (I was to learn later that the psychologists have described it as ‘fear spread thinly.’) There was no reason to feel worried about anything, after all I still had my job and if I didn’t like the sound of things I could just say “Thank you for your time,” and walk away, but there I was following Mr. O’Rourke down this interminably long echoing, empty and dismal corridor with my heart in my mouth as if I were a condemned man about to face the gallows.

After we had gone quite a distance we passed a long notice board with a florescent strip light flickering above it. Later, during my training, I and all the other students would come to know this notice board well. Sometimes it would bring us good news, sometimes bad, as we looked for our next ward placement, or to find out who would be our companion whilst on night duty, and many of other the things that would affect our lives, it would sometimes tell us things that would make us happy, but quite often it said things that made us sad.

Mr. O’Rourke suddenly took a left turn, drew a heavy bunch of keys attached to a chain from his pocket and unlocked one of four doors situated in a dark alcove.

"Come on in, this is the nursing office where all the real work takes place," he said with a grin. I think he realised how I was feeling and was trying to be reassuring.

He allowed me to go in ahead of him, and then closed the door behind us. Again, like the notice board this would be a place that I would know in the future, some times my experiences in that office would be pleasant, but occasionally they would, I'm afraid, be rather less than enjoyable.

As I said earlier I remember little of the conversation, only that I was concerned about money, because as a student I would be taking a forty percent drop in wages. He was able to give me the information that I needed, which wasn't reassuring, but as it happens only a few months after I started nurse training we had a very good pay rise and another one a couple of years, or so later that made things a lot easier for the struggling nurse.

No one was well off in those days, because nursing was mainly a female profession and hadn't at that time got equal pay rights. As a result, for many years nurses were poorly paid. The job was looked upon as a vocation, a calling, 'helping mankind.' I wonder if that's why so many families worked in psychiatric hospitals, generations of them in some cases. Perhaps if they all worked together and were able to obtain a hospital house, they may have been able to have lived reasonably well, especially as they would be able to use a lot of the facilities available within the hospital grounds.

I wasn't able at the time, as far as I can remember to take a look around any of the wards, as it was the time of day when they were busy getting ready for the night staff to come on duty. If I'd had the opportunity to see the hospital properly I think I would have made a hasty retreat, but as it was, that summers evening in 1974 I took my leave of Mr. O'Rourke, carrying in my hand an application form for the post of nursing assistant, with a promise that another one enabling me to apply for nurse training would soon be in the post.

I don't recall my feelings as I left him, but something in our conversation must have persuaded me that I was taking the right step.

Would I live to regret it?

As I drove away I felt that this was the right move to make, but later I would realise that I should have done my research more thoroughly. However, even though I'm glad that I took the decision to do my training, if I'd known that evening how the next couple of encounters with the hospital would turn out, I most certainly wouldn't have gone into psychiatric nursing as a profession.

Chapter two.

"What do you really think, Bev?" I asked my wife while cleaning off the saliva from one of the kitchen cupboard doors. Sheba, our dog, a boxer had shaken her head violently, as dogs do and had left her trademark all over the place.

"You've asked me a hundred times, Robert and I've told you, I don't mind as long as there's enough money coming in to feed us. You must do as you want." She replied wearily.

Beverly and I had been married since we were eighteen and she was really easy going, but at that moment in time I didn't want 'easy going', I wanted to know what she really thought was the best thing to do. Should I go for a job that was going to leave us poverty stricken, but give me some sort of satisfaction, or should I continue with the comfortable, yet somehow meaningless way of life that I had now. I wanted her to tell me that it was a good thing to go into nursing so, I suppose, secretly I could blame her if things weren't what I expected. On the other hand if she were to say she didn't want to make the sacrifice involved, at least I hadn't made the decision and I could always hold a self pitying resentment against her for stopping me from doing what I really wanted to do!

A nursing officer told me not so long ago,

"There are leaders and followers in this world Robert, and you, I'm afraid to say are a follower."

I must admit this hurt me; after all I had risen to the dizzy heights of being a charge nurse by then, yet really I knew he was right. I didn't like making life-changing decisions. I'd rather Bev did it with me and with her taking the leading role just in case I made a major mistake; it was so much easier that way. I'd never been very brave, I wasn't the officer material that would have led the charge in the trenches during the First World War, pistol in hand, shouting

"Come on lads, over the top!"

I was more like a common soldier who would pretend to be tying his shoe lace while the others went over first, hoping that the danger would be past by the time he made his appearance.

"Ok. if your going to take the middle of the road approach, I suppose I'll make the decision and go for it then," I told her unconvincingly.

"Anyway I suppose if things become a bit sticky your dad'll always help us out a bit," I said with a secret hope that she'd protest at this and open it all up again, but she didn't.

The whole thing was so difficult. I was ambivalent, I'd had sleepless nights and discussed it over and over again, but when all was said and done, despite my fears I thought I ought to send my application in.

So I filled in the forms and sent them off, then confided in a few people what I was planning to do. Most of my family and the few friends that I had told, thought that I was crazy for taking such a drop in wages to do a job which some warned me wasn't as glamorous as the advertising literature seemed to make it appear.

I must admit that I was, to say the least, feeling rather shaky about it all, especially as several times in the week my delivery route took me past St. Andrews which was the name of the hospital I was trying to get into and although I had never taken much notice before, from the road stretching my neck on every occasion I passed, I could see that it was a huge complex of buildings covering several acres, looking to me then huge and foreboding. There was a wall and there were railings around much of it, but in places it was more open for access, unlike years ago when it was apparently fully enclosed and in fact more or less self sufficient.

In the old days, long before my time it had had a farm and a dairy, also a piggery and stables for the horses that worked on the farm and no doubt, housing for the staff that worked with the horses that were used before the advent of the tractor.

A lot of the patients had worked on the farm, and in these days when we think of someone with a mental illness we may not understand how that many of the them under the old system, before my time, used to get up at the crack of dawn to milk the cows, or feed the pigs and chickens etc. and apparently they seemed to have actually enjoyed it. It gave them a point to their lives that they may never had been able to fulfil outside of the hospital due to their mental state.

Now of course all this has gone and we would regard such a regime and system as exploitation of the mentally ill. Perhaps there is a lot in that, but I can't help but think that maybe we've thrown the baby out with the bathwater.

I believe that not too long before I started working there most of the staff had lived in the hospital grounds, and there was even a huge church where both staff and patients were, I was later told, obliged to attend on a Sunday, the Roman Catholic's being allowed to travel into town about four miles away to attend mass. Only around twenty years before I was to grace the place with my presence, to become a male attendant, as they were then known, one had to be able to play a decent game of football, or cricket, and the staff at various hospitals would compete not only in their own grounds, but at other venues too.

Our own hospital had a football field and a cricket pitch, as well as an immaculately kept bowling green. The requirement that made it necessary in those bygone days to undertake nurse training was that one had to be keen on sport. That would have precluded me, as I had always had a strong aversion to the game of football and other such sports, partly because my dad had more than encouraged me, but in fact, rather forced me to go out with my football and seek a game with a few of the local lads because, I suppose it would render me more manly in his eyes.

Oh, how I hated football! In fact I was happier reading a book, or even skipping, or perhaps playing hopscotch in the street with the girls next door, much to dads consternation.

"Why aren't you in the field with a ball instead of being stuck in here on a nice day like this?" He'd demand, after arriving home from work unexpectedly.

The disappointment in his tone was always very evident to me. Immediately he'd make me go trudging up to the field at the top of the road to seek out enthusiastic football players.

Then of course there was cricket; to this day I can't understand the rules and although there's something very nice and English about seeing a cricket match taking place on a village green, I have to confess I really can't muster any interest in the game. Sorry, any cricket fans that may be reading this! Perhaps that's because of a day that sticks in my mind when I was helping my dad on his allotment.

Seeing there were some boys playing cricket nearby he told me,

"Go over and ask if I can play with them."

To my relief, when I went and asked to join them they said 'No.'

I told my dad that they didn't want me to play with them, but instead of saying 'ok,' the reply was,

"Go back and tell them that you're going to play with them whether they like it or not.

"Dad, I can't say that," I protested, feebly.

"If you don't I'll give you a clip across the ear," he told me in no uncertain terms.

In my days it wasn't unusual for parents, or teachers, especially teachers, to smack a child around the head, sometimes so violently, that in my case, at least it would make my ears ring. So obediently I went back to the lads and relayed dads message. As a result of my conversation with them I nearly got beaten up. Such were the methods dad used to make me more manly!

Anyway back to the hospital.

Basically it had been like a self contained little village, where I imagine everyone knew everyone else and every one did everything together, to some extent at least. Even in my day there was a nurses home where female nurses had one floor and males another, and ne'er the twain would meet, theoretically! There was a staff canteen and a kitchen and a huge dining room and an equally massive sitting room in the nurses home where, off duty, staff, whether caterers or nurses, or whoever, would meet up. There was also a theatre where the staff would perform for the patients and the staffs relatives, and in fact even in my time once a year there would be a pantomime, which the leading members of the theatre group would always be trying to press gang their colleagues into taking part. I, fortunately always managed to escape their net, or perhaps they didn't think that I was good enough!

I didn't know all about this at the time of my application of course. All I knew was that the hospital looked so big that I was sure that there would be hundreds of people working there and, being rather shy I was a little nervous about whether or not I would fit in and be accepted. I still hadn't given up on being super-nurse of course, but in the back of my mind I knew that it would probably take a little more time than I had originally anticipated.

A couple of weeks after sending in the application forms I received a letter asking me if I would attend for interview at the nursing school within the hospital grounds, at two o clock the next Thursday. That was my busiest day at work and my delivery round was fifteen miles away, I wasn't sure that I would make it on time, but I daren't ask my boss for the time off as he would have probably told me that if I wanted another job I could relinquish this one forthwith, or words to that effect. If anyone wanted to attend for an interview in those days it was expected that they would do it in their own time!

Fearful, yet excited, I took the bull by the horns and replied that I would be very pleased to attend.

I could hardly believe it, although I finished my deliveries early on that day due to my rushing around like a crazy man, I was held up on the way back into town by a minor car crash. The hospital was on one side of town and I was on the other. As soon as I could, I put my foot down on the accelerator and drove as fast as my poor old van would go, doing a detour so as to avoid the town centre.

I finally arrived, but despite my most valiant efforts I was ten minutes late.

The receptionist told me unsympathetically,

"Sorry dear, but I can't let you go in, you're too late, you should have been here on time."

Out of character, I exploded!

"Just a minute! I've rushed here as fast as possible, everything was against me, it's not my fault and I'm not going away until I've had the chance to apply for this job."

The suitably chastened receptionist left her little cubicle, excusing herself and, a couple of minutes later a familiar and friendly face appeared, a short tubby man with rosy cheeks and with a smile that I remembered from years ago. I recalled even at this moment that that smile never seemed to leave his face.

I had known Rees on and off for about seven years, whilst he was a theological student at the college close to where I worked as an assistant in a hardware shop, during my late teens. I often had to deliver various things to the college and bumped into Rees on many occasions, we used to discuss theological matters and mostly disagree during our encounters. Although I couldn't say that he was a friend, we had known each other very well, in fact he had even gone on to be the curate at the church on the estate where I lived. He was just the person that I needed at this moment in time, because it just so happened that he was one of the tutors in the nurse training school and he had given up theology to make a career in the caring profession.

"Hurry up, I think you still might have time." He said hurriedly, gasping for breath, as he had obviously been asked most urgently to attend to this troublesome man at reception.

Despite his breathlessness he continued to wear his warm smile.

I needed no second bidding and followed him into a large room full of desks and chairs, where sat a number of people in studious silence, obviously there was an exam going on. Rees quickly motioned to me to be seated at the only empty desk.

He placed an envelope before me and whispered,

"You have ten minutes, hurry up." Then he immediately left the room.

An exam? I was absolutely useless at exams. The last one I remember taking was during my final year at secondary school. The subject was maths and my best friend sat next to me and copied my answers. I came last and he, second to last, he obviously made a mistake! Perhaps there's a moral in there somewhere.

I had been to what was probably the worst school in town, we didn't even have the opportunity to do GCEs there. If you were considered bright enough for higher education you were sent to the local grammar school to finish your education there. As for myself, well I didn't exactly shine in the academic area, in fact I spent most of my time messing around and playing the teachers up. The cane, the slipper and the strap were no strangers to me and were often felt on various tender parts of my anatomy! Mind you I have to say, I loved my schooldays immensely; I didn't learn much it's true, but I enjoyed myself tremendously.

When, on the last day of the last term at school all the fourth year lads were throwing their caps into the air in jubilation, shouting, "Hurray!" because it was all over for them. I was sad and downhearted.

Not only would I have to get a job now, but also I'd have to leave all these people behind, not just my friends, but also my teachers. In a funny sort of way I cared for them, despite their occasional brutality. And for a number of years afterwards I made nostalgic trips back to visit my old teachers, which must have been very boring and inconvenient to them, as they tried to conduct their lessons with me getting in the way.

Back to the exam!

It hadn't dawned upon me up to that point in the process that if I were going to apply for nurse training, and if I were to be a student nurse, I would probably have to take the odd exam, or two and also to attend a great many lectures. As it turned out, though this wasn't an exam, but an aptitude test; the typical question being

'If farmer Giles has ten cows and one goes walkabouts, another gets savaged by a wolf, but in the meantime three give birth, how many cows would farmer Giles have at the end of the day?'

Well I did my best and completed all the questions, before the man who sat watching us throughout picked up his little hand bell and called an end to the proceedings.

Everyone sat in silence, as one by one after the aptitude test we were called out of the room by Rees, to be led into another room for our formal interview. Rees, of course was there, but so too was another welsh man who, having introduced himself as Bill Jones I felt certain was a friend of my auntie. Being impetuous as I was, I asked him straight away if he knew her, as she was the one who had recommended that I apply for training. Immediately the interview got off to a good start. I was asked the usual questions like,

'Why do you want to do nursing?' and,

'What can you offer the patients here?' etc, etc.

I got through it the best way I could and seemed to have made a reasonable impression.

After a few minutes I was striding out of the room, with the promise that as long as my test was ok. I would be given a place on the next course, which was to commence in just a few weeks time.

I was ecstatic, and almost floated back to my car, and was talking to myself in excitement all the way home. People who drove past me probably thought that I was mad, but I was in the seventh heaven. All I had to do now was to await the outcome of my exam.

A number of years later Bill Jones and I would work together on night duty after, he had relinquished his post as a nursing officer to become a charge nurse, We became good friends and I was able, after some hesitation to call him by his first name, which to me was extremely difficult, being used to only using surnames with the majority of the senior staff. The reason why he and so many others worked night duty during their final years of service was that their pensions would be greatly improved, due to the extra duty payments they received for working unsociable hours.

Chapter 3.

It wasn't many days before I received a letter through the post telling me that I had been successful in my interview and had passed the test. I now was to become a student nurse with a two-week introductory period as a nursing assistant. I was asked to start in the third week of September, presenting myself for duty at Devon ward on a Monday at two o' clock.

Despite my nervousness at what lay ahead I, nevertheless gave my notice in at work. Needless to say everyone voiced their disappointment at my leaving, or warned me of their concerns that by becoming a mental nurse I might in fact become one of the patients myself someday. Even, Jeff with whom I had never got on very well and I suspected was being insincere when he wished me all the best for the future, appeared to be sad to see me go, but that is always the same in any firm, you think they're going to miss you, then two weeks later they can barely remember your name!

'Boss,' that was what we called the manager of the firm, told me that if it didn't work out, there was always a job waiting for me. I didn't really believe him because I knew that at the wages he was offering he would fill my position within a few days, nevertheless it was nice to hear him say it.

The two younger members of staff with whom I had occasionally worked in the warehouse suggested that by becoming a nurse I was probably gay. Actually they didn't use the word 'gay,' but a rather more insulting expression, (I don't think that the word gay was used in the context that we use it today anyway.) There was no such thing as political correctness in those days, so it wasn't as unusual as it is now to hear such expressions bandied about in an insulting and hurtful way.

"Don't be a plonker Robert!" Gary, one of the lads shouted from the top of a stack of boxes, before climbing onto the pallet resting on the prongs of the forklift truck, then waiting for me to let him down. "You'll turn into one of the inmates before the years out."

It was his last desperate attempt to save me from a terrible mistake, or so he thought and I had to admit I was a little afraid of that myself.

In my teens I'd known a lad who'd worked up at the hospital, but he'd given the job up after a little while. I was a little wary of him and always kept my distance. He seemed a bit odd to me and I never got too friendly with him, just in case he had contracted a mental illness. I know this all sounds silly and naïve, but youth and ignorance are my only excuse.

Nevertheless despite all of this I continued on my path of possible self-destruction. I worked my week's notice trying to look as manly as possible while in the warehouse, so the lads believed that I was 'normal,' then after having had a few days off as a sort of holiday, the time came around for me to present myself at the hospital.

Now I was nervous and wished that I hadn't started all this. I wished that I had opted for the status quo, but that afternoon shortly before two pm. I found myself standing in front of the large wooden door of Devon ward.

I was anxious, to say the least as I pressed the large doorbell which was adjacent to the great big painted door that had probably been there for a hundred and fifty years. I wondered what stories it could tell, as I waited in fearful anticipation of what was beyond. I still had in my mind that whatever lay ahead, I was there for a purpose and my presence would make a difference to the people on that ward.

Eventually I heard the click clack of a woman's shoes; I heard the key turning slowly in the lock and the door was opened by a woman of about forty, who was very stout and very foreboding.

“Yes?” was all that she said.

“I’m Robert Panton and I’m your new nurse,” I said quickly and nervously.

I didn’t like the look of her, she had a squint and I frankly confess that I didn’t know which eye to look into, and anyway I didn’t like her demeanour, after all I had come to help people, not to be intimidated.

I learned later that this was Lorna, the ward orderly and that she had once been a patient herself. What she was she couldn’t help, but at that time I was very unlearned in the things of the psychiatric world and I resented her, not only at the very beginning for not being more welcoming, but afterwards, as I encountered her unwanted behaviour.

For instance there were several times while she was mopping the day room floor and, because I would be sent off the ward on an errand, or I had to go to see to a patient I was forced to walk across that nice clean, wet floor. How she would shout at me, despite my protests that I didn’t have any other choice. Even when I tip toed and skirted around the edges she shouted loud and venomous insults at me.

The worst thing was that she had no appreciation of classical music, which I was then starting to enjoy.

One morning I was looking through a pile of records having been asked by the charge nurse to put some music on for the patients, I found an LP. of Beethoven's fifth piano concerto, which up until then I had never heard. The first movement played itself through without comment, or incident, but just as the second movement was getting under way and I was melting at the sheer beauty of it, (oblivious as to whether, or not the patients were enjoying it) out came Lorna from the kitchen, in a fume,

"I've heard enough of that rubbish. Turn it off now, or I'll break the record over your head!" She shouted.

I could see that she was serious and looking around at the other staff members faces I knew by their expressions that I had better comply.

Later when I understood her better I was ashamed of my hidden, though real hostility towards her, not realising that many of the staff made allowances for her because they knew of Lorna's previous psychiatric history. It was years before I heard the complete recording of Beethoven's fifth piano concerto, but to this day it is one of my favourite classical works and have it written into my will that I would like the second movement played as my coffin is carried down the aisle.

On that first encounter with Lorna she led me through the large dayroom without speaking a word, her shoes echoing on the tiled floor. Coming to the ward office she stopped and knocked on the closed door and strode off again in the direction of the ward kitchen without a word, leaving me standing there feeling foolish waiting for goodness knows who, to greet me. As I looked around I was horrified, nothing could have prepared me for what I would see in the ward day room, with its adjacent dining room.

The room was large and light enough, with its high ceiling and windows to three sides, but it was the occupants of the room that held my attention. I know that I was probably naïve not to have known, but when I saw all those old men either wandering around aimlessly, or sitting staring at nothing, or groaning and crying out to who knows who, or what, it was as if my whole world was shaken.

What had I come to? This wasn't at all what I had expected.

It was what was known as a geriatric ward and (now known as Care of the Elderly Mentally Ill.) stupid and unforgivable as it may seem, I had no idea that there were such people as geriatrics, who suffered with dementia. Naïve in the extreme, I'd never considered that there could be such people in a mental hospital. I know that at the age of twenty-five it seems incredible, but it's true. I felt as if I wanted to disappear.

And the smell! It wasn't what I associated with a hospital.

To be honest the smell of a general hospital in those days was of ether, which though unpleasant, was a clean smell. Devon ward wasn't like that at all. Later I would try to analyse it. Was it the smoking that did it, or the incontinent patients, or the food they served up? I don't know; it was certainly clean enough. Whatever I felt about Lorna she was always dusting and mopping, or doing something to enhance the cleanliness of her ward, in fact she had a very busy life, as she was also responsible for the ward kitchen.

Within a couple of minutes, during which time I was wondering how I could escape from this nightmarish situation, a small, slightly built Asian man opened the door. Introducing himself as Frank, he asked me to come into the small ward office, which contained a desk, a few filing cabinets and three or four chairs.

"I'm sorry," he said in a thick Indian sounding accent. "But, I have to go to a meeting, if you put one of these white coats on," pointing to a number of rather grubby looking articles that hung on the back of the door.

"You can go and help out with the toileting. Tomorrow I'll send you down to the sewing room to be fitted up with a suit and some white coats of your own."

I thanked him and found myself a reasonable coat then left the office. Outside I stood there, not knowing what to do next.

Suddenly I heard a voice calling out shrilly. "Come on, come on, come on. I'm wet, wet, wet, wet, wet!"

Looking in the direction of this, which was to me a strange sounding voice, I saw a very small man with a bald head, and whose face seemed to be covered in dandruff, he was around eighty years of age.

"Give us a hand love." A female nurse, whom I hadn't noticed sitting nearby, said to me as she got up out of her seat.

"I'll do what I can," I replied, "but I'm afraid that I've only just started and don't know what I'm supposed to do."

"Oh don't worry about that we all have to start somewhere, you'll soon get the hang of it. This is Billy," she pointed to the patient in question, "When he's wet you can be sure that a lot of the others will be too, and as you can see, he makes a bit of a fuss about it."

I learned that Billy had been a postman, cycling around the remote parts of the county. To me it seemed incredible that someone in this present condition could have been responsible enough to have delivered the post.

Little by little Kat showed me the procedure for changing an incontinent patient and she also helped me to see that what I saw now in these people wasn't what they were years ago. In their time they had been able, like myself to hold a job down, but what had happened to them came unexpectedly and was painful not only to them, but also to their families.

As we talked we had to meet the need in hand, and as Billy couldn't stand and bear his own weight we had to get either side of him and lift him bodily off of his seat, while another nurse, a student named Maurice pulled off his pyjama bottoms, then pulled another pair up to his waist, following that he swiftly removed the wet drawer sheet beneath Billy and replaced it with a clean one. A blanket was then placed around his legs to keep him warm, after Kat had given him a quick kiss to the top of his bald scaly head, we moved on to the next patient.

Years later I would have given any nurses under my authority, a good dressing down if they had done things this way, but at that time there were no hoists, no pads and no screens available to give the patient privacy whilst doing this type of care. It was quite simply how it was done, not only on this ward, but throughout the hospital. No washing, no explanation of the procedure to the patient, no thoughts about personal dignity, just a rush job before moving on to the next one in the line, just like a conveyor belt.

After we had finished with the incontinent patients we moved on to "toileting" the more able and mobile ones. These men wore ordinary daytime clothing, not pyjamas. True much of their attire was ill fitting, but at least they looked presentable.

I was assigned to Tom, a thin agitated man of around seventy, who was unwilling to leave his seat, but Maurice who was a well-built young man lifted him up, and although Tom struggled he gave him into my care. I instinctively placed my right arm around his waist and held his left hand in mine, attempting to reassure him as I held him up and led him to the toilet. I soon realised that he wasn't listening to me; in fact he was muttering something indiscernible under his breath as I led him to the toilet block.

"Try and use the toilet, Tom," I urged, hopefully.

Tom continued muttering and staring ahead into space. I realised that he couldn't comprehend and so I unzipped his flies and much against my will, and very uncomfortably, I took out his penis; with the toilet before him I thought that he would certainly use it, after all he must have done it hundreds of thousands of times before during his lifetime: but no, nothing! What should I do? I waited and waited and encouraged and pleaded, but I had failed, how could I take him back and tell the others that he hadn't performed? By this time I felt the perspiration forming on my brow, but it was useless, we had been there for ten minutes, and he hadn't passed even a drop of urine.

Kat intervened,

"Don't worry love it often happens, why do you think so many of them are in pyjamas? Penny to a pound that he'll do it in his trousers before tea time."

I was relieved, (excuse the pun) at least it felt as though I hadn't failed after all. I was given another patient to toilet within a couple of minutes and then another after that, thankfully they both performed the required task. Boy, was I thankful when I was told that it was time for a cup of tea!

How welcome these tea/coffee breaks were over the next couple of weeks; after then hopefully, when I had completed my six weeks training course in the PTS. (Preliminary training school,) I would be given a placement on the sort of ward I had been expecting, i.e. an acute admission ward. Not that at that time I knew that they were called by that name, nor had I given much thought to the fact that the training course took three years and I would have to serve my time on many different wards and come across a wide variety of mental illnesses. All this would be in the future, and when inevitably the other staff members questioned me about how I liked it so far and why had I wanted to be a psychiatric nurse, I tried hard not to show much of the bitter disappointment that I felt after only a couple of hours in the job.

They were a friendly bunch on the whole, apart from the staff nurse a stout, balding man of about thirty or so who, one of the nursing assistants discretely told me later was gay, apparently his ex partner worked on night duty on Devon ward.

"And don't burst into a fit of laughter if he comes into work one day wearing a wig, or he'll make the rest of your time here a misery," she whispered, with a big grin on her face.

The tea break, was taken in the day room so as to observe the patients and indeed we often had one or two of them sitting with us, or annoyingly wandering around the table where we sat. During this twenty minutes respite I asked a lot of questions, and found that this was a relatively small ward of twenty four patients, each of whom were highly dependant in one way or another.

There were usually six staff on duty on each shift, consisting normally, of a charge nurse, staff nurse, in our case it was Henry, then possibly, an S.E.N. (state enrolled nurse) and a student, or two, with the numbers being made up with the nursing assistants. The S.E.N. was often somebody who had either undergone two years training, or had been given the grade because they had worked as a nursing auxiliary for many years. I suppose it was a recognition of their loyalty over a long period of time. Each grade was recognised among the females, at least by the colour of the band, or bands on their caps. With the male staff there didn't seem to be any distinguishing features in our particular hospital.

"Right then, this wont do; work calls," Maurice said after about twenty minutes.

Getting up out of his seat he motioned to me to follow him. He led the way to the top end of the ward and through a pair of double doors into the dormitory, where lined up on either side were beds, most of which had what are now known as safety rails, but were then called cot sides.

I stood one side of each of the beds and Maurice the other side, as he trained me in the art of turning down the bed covers ready for the later task of putting the patients to bed. I said that it was an art form and indeed it was, as were lots of things in the dormitories. The beds, which of course had been made meticulously using hospital corners, had to be turned down so that the upper sheet formed a 'v' shape and all the beds had to be uniform and be exactly spaced apart so that if the nursing officer happened to pass by he, or she would be satisfied with what they saw.

"Have you been shown around the fire points yet?" Asked Maurice, probably already knowing the answer."

"No, I haven't even seen a lot of the ward at all," I answered frankly.

"Well someone's been a bit naughty. In the absence of the charge nurse Harry should have given you a guided tour. Never mind," he said, as we brought the trolley of linen and towels out of the sluice ready for the night staff. "Its too late now, I'll have a word with him and it'll have to be done tomorrow, come on, meal time is next on the agenda."

I followed him back into the day room where in our absence the tables had been laid for the evening meal. Some of the patients made their own way to their usual tables, others needed help. There were about half a dozen that stayed in their seats and portable tables were brought to them. These patients were what were known as 'the babies,' they needed a lot of assistance with feeding themselves. In fact some of them couldn't do anything at all without a great deal of physical intervention from the nursing staff in every area of their sad lives.

It was messy at mealtimes, but somehow very rewarding if you were assigned to a couple of patients who were totally reliant upon you for their food.

There was one old chap, Harry who as I tried to spoon feed him his meal that evening, kept sticking his rather large tongue out just as I was about to put the food in, he was on a soft diet, because he was a choking risk, so as he knocked the food off the spoon it splattered down onto the gravy, which in turn splattered my already grubby white coat: I now knew why I needed one!

"Don't worry love, if you can't get him to eat it, I'll find him a 'Build up' and you can give him it out of a feeder cup, some days he's better than others," Kat said kindly, watching my miserable failure, much to my embarrassment.

A few moments later she appeared with a covered plastic cup that had a spout at the end that I could place in the side of the patients mouth out of the way of his tongue; success at last!

While all this was going on Frank and Henry were giving the medicines out to various patients, after this Frank called me into his office and apologised for not being there earlier to show me around and tell me about the ward.

"But, tomorrow I'll make it up to you, the afternoon shift starts at a quarter to one; today was your first day so we let you off lightly and allowed you to start late. As soon as I've received the handover from the morning staff tomorrow afternoon I'll have a chat with you. I'm not going to ask you how you feel about things now, because it'll all seem a bit overwhelming, but tomorrow things will, I promise you seem a little better, I know from my own experience."

It seemed obvious to me that Henry, or Maurice, or Kat had spoken to him during the shift and told him how green I was!

I thanked him, as I left the office to see what was expected of me next. Kat collared me as I stepped into the ward,

"Would you help me to get some of the babies to bed, please Robert," she asked, as she pushed a wheelchair before her.

I readily agreed, following her lead.

First into the wheelchair was Billy, who was quickly taken through to one of the beds lining the left hand side of the dormitory. With some difficulty we lifted him up onto the bed whilst removing his pyjama bottoms. Next the trolley containing a jug of hot water, the flannels and the towels was drawn on it's wheels to a convenient place nearby and Kat gave Billy a wash around his lower parts, showered some talcum powder onto the area after drying, and after pulling a doubled up drawer sheet between his legs, we pulled his bed covers up over him. Finally she showed me how to work the antiquated cot sides, once satisfied that they were properly in place she quickly gave him a kiss on his cheek, oblivious to his scaly skin, and said goodnight. In all this Billy never uttered a sound, or showed the slightest resistance to what was being done to him.

On then to the next patient, and what a difference, this was Ralph, a big powerful man who could become very emotional and would begin to cry like a baby and resist all intervention at times. The way around this during the day was to bribe him with a cigarette, but as there was no smoking in the dormitory, things could become very difficult, sometimes requiring three nurses to assist.

That night things were going on well, as he was already wandering around the ward and only needed steering in the right direction. Once at his bed however, he objected strongly to being stripped of his pyjama bottoms and began to let out some very loud cries of

"Wont do it! Wont do it!" much to my consternation. He began to physically resist our intervention and Frank came out of his office to help us out. I thought Kat was good, but Frank with his quiet voice soon, to my amazement had Ralph eating out of his hand, I'm not sure how he did it, but there was something magical about the way he had diffused the situation. Ralph did refuse a draw sheet between his legs, (these by the way were placed there in a vain attempt to prevent the whole bed becoming saturated in the sure event of urinary incontinence) but he climbed into bed like a lamb and settled down for sleep immediately.

By the time we had finished with Ralph the majority of the so-called babies had been put to bed by the other staff.

"I think you can go home now Robert," Frank said, after assuring himself that much of the work had been done.

"It's been a tiring day and you'll need to get a good nights sleep ready for tomorrow."

Thanking him I dashed into the office before he changed his mind, took off my white coat and said a hasty farewell to everyone and was let out of the locked door. It was eight thirty, half an hour before the end of the shift. Oh, how lovely the evening seemed to be outside, all that wonderful fresh air!

Chapter 4

The next day I arrived promptly for my second shift. I'd had a sleepless night and waiting for the afternoon to come around, I felt worried and miserable. It didn't seem natural to me to be working late shifts, and then early shifts and it took me some time to get into the swing of it. On top of this I kept on feeling depressed, thinking about those poor old men, who through no fault of their own had landed in what must have appeared to them to be some sort of nightmare, that's providing of course they could understand their situation at all.

Nevertheless I rang the doorbell of Devon ward and was let in by one of the morning shift. Handover was going on, so the staff who weren't involved were sitting having a drink, interfered with, as usual by some of the more mobile of the patients. I wish I could really convey what it was like in those early days of working in psychiatry.

Alzheimer's wasn't a term that was used, only dementia. There were two types I was to learn later; one was due to hardening of the arteries (that was the explanation students were given,) and the other was organic. Of course, then I didn't know the difference, all I knew was that there was a ward full of old men who weren't in control of their faculties.

"He's confused," I was told, but that didn't fit into my idea of confusion.

Nonetheless everyone was very pleasant. Both morning and afternoon staff sat around the table, and appeared to me to be at odds with the tragic circumstances of the patients. The staff appeared so unconcerned and joked with one another, or talked about their every day lives, whereas I couldn't help but feel depressed by it all!

The staff of course wanted to know all about me and I told them something about myself. Kat, who to me was a crutch the day before, was off duty that day, but I met several others of the nursing assistants, they were all very nice and made me feel a little more relaxed. Maurice, the student, asked me to help him with some toilet training.

Some of the patients weren't totally incontinent and if they were taken to the toilet regularly they would often respond favourably. To prevent them from deteriorating in this area they were 'toileted' every few hours. One of these was Wilf who, with a little assistance was able to make his way to the toilet.

I took him, as requested and lo and behold, he performed, I felt elated, for once I had done something unaided, and done it right! The only words I could get out of him though, as I attempted to talk with him was,

"Aye. Aye." Nothing else.

I wanted so much to have a rational conversation, to find out where he had come from, what he had done for a living. Was he married, did he have any children? All I got was "Aye!"

For quite a time after the morning staff had left we continued toileting and changing the patients, then I was summoned to the office by Frank. He was kindness itself. Somehow he'd sensed that the first day hadn't been all that I'd expected.

"Robert," he said, in his thick Indian accent.

"When I came from India to do my general nurse training, it was all that I had imagined, but when, I'd finished there I decided to do my psychiatric nurse training, I could hardly believe my eyes. Not only were the type of patient not what I had quite expected, but also the way they were looked upon and treated, even sometimes by the staff that were caring for them was undesirable to my way of thinking. I wanted to try and make the lives of the patients on this ward at the very least comfortable. I know that we can't do away with their dementia, but we can make their lives a little more bearable. I believe that's what you'd want, isn't it?"

He looked at me and didn't speak again, obviously wanting me to agree to his desires for his patients, knowing, of course that I would really, how could it be otherwise? (I learned later that this little pep talk in the office was always procedure for a new member of staff, and how brilliant, I thought when I understood his tactics!) I did agree that I wanted to do my best and that I had come into the job for that reason, I didn't however tell him all that was on my heart.

When Frank was satisfied that I was, as it were, on his side, he allowed me to leave the office, with the promise that he would help me all he could to learn how to care for patients in a way that was acceptable, especially in the next two weeks before I began my training. After his little speech, much to my relief he gave me a key to the ward; it felt much better to be able to come and go without having to rely on someone else to open the door.

As I emerged from the office Maurice was waiting eagerly for me.

"What did he say?" he asked in anticipation.

I told him the gist of the conversation.

"I knew it!" he exclaimed, "He said the same to me when I first started. Apparently when he came to St. Andrews he was so shocked by what he saw on the geriatric wards that he promised himself that he would try to make things better. It's not that all the wards are bad, its just Frank. He feels that they should be better, Devon isn't a pleasant ward to work on, that's for certain, but with Frank as the charge nurse, there's one thing for sure, you'll get some good training here."

"You probably don't realise," he went on, but this is my last placement. When you are in your final year you can choose where you would like to end up; I chose here, just because I have so much respect for Frank. As for Henry, the reason he's so miserable is because he doesn't like it; he prefers the old way of treating the patients as if they are just there to meet his need to earn a wage, but with Frank it's a passion. He wants the patients to feel as if they really matter. I know that things aren't perfect, but Frank has made things a lot better than they were."

"Anyway I've been asked by Henry to give you a guided tour of the ward, and then you have to go and get measured up for a suit. Oh, and by the way, don't lose your key or you'll have to pay ten pounds out for another one!"

I followed him around, as he showed me the fire points and fire doors and then on into the sluice, where he told me all about how the sterilisation of the bedpans and urine bottles was done.

"At the weekend it will be your job, on any ward that you're on as a first year student to clean the sluice out, and woe betide you if it isn't perfect. Most sisters and charge nurses are really fussy about their sluices, but don't worry about it you'll be shown what's expected of you."

The tour of the ward took about fifteen minutes, after which I was directed up to the sewing room.

I walked slowly through the bare, dingy, echoing corridors feeling shy and conspicuous as I passed various nurses, some alone, and others in groups, occasionally someone without a uniform would stride by me. One or two looked quite officious to my way of thinking, so I averted my eyes as they walked on by. Then I saw a middle-aged man, thin and stooping, with saliva dribbling out of his mouth as he shuffled along. I didn't feel very encouraged by this, but by now I was beginning to realise that things weren't how I had imagined them to be anyway.

Eventually I reach my destination and knocked on the door, I was let in by a very friendly lady who introduced me to a smartly dressed gentleman who, within a few minutes had measured me up for a suit; well two suits actually, one to wear and another in reserve for when the first needed to be cleaned. Oddly enough, I had worked at a local tailors when in my teens, which had supplied many of the suits for the male nurses at St. Andrews, little did I know that one day I would be fitted out with one of them myself.

After I had been measured and had chosen the style from a few very limited options I was given a pile of new white coats, which I carried back to the ward, feeling a strange mixture of pride having now obtained my own coats and so feeling a little more like a real nurse, yet on the other hand regretting that I had started the whole thing in the first place; still time would tell.

'If I really don't like it here,' I thought, 'I can always get a job out in the real world again.' I knew that I wouldn't though; I'd be too ashamed of having started something that I couldn't finish.

Back on the ward after having deposited my coats in the office and putting one of them on, I went to help with the toileting. Susan, a health care assistant who hadn't been on duty the day before showed me how to empty a catheter into a bottle, as I hadn't seen anyone with a catheter before. There wasn't a catheter bag just a tube coming out of the patients penis, which to me didn't seem odd at the time, only later would I know better. I asked her why it was that all the incontinent patients didn't have one, as it seemed a much better idea than their wetting themselves every few hours. She explained that, because of the risk of infection only those with retention of urine could have a catheter fitted and that was why a lot of patients were taken to the toilet regularly, trying to keep them continent. I found this and many other things that I encountered over the next couple of weeks fascinating. It wasn't necessary to enjoy the work I suppose, to find it interesting.

The shift sped by that day and before I realised it, it was evening. I was spared the job of getting the less able patients into bed for the night staff, as staff nurse Henry, who seemed to be in a brighter mood that day called me into the clinic, which was always kept locked, so it was the first time I'd seen inside it

It was quite a small room and clean looking, not that the rest of the ward wasn't in good order, it was just that with all the packets of sterile dressings and packs of equally sterile instruments stacked neatly on shelves, and with the immaculately clean medicine trolley the room seemed quite glowing to me.

"This is my little kingdom," Henry said quite proudly.

"Other people come in here of course, but I like to keep it nice and tidy and to be quite honest prefer to spend as much time in here as I can, away from that lot." He gestured towards the patients.

I asked him why he stayed in nursing if he didn't want to be with the patients. His reply to me was that his mum and dad were nurses, and having been brought up within the hospital grounds it seemed quite natural to follow in his parent's footsteps.

"But if you don't like it, why don't you do something else?" I asked.

"For one very good reason," he replied, candidly, "I can retire at fifty five on a reasonable pension and really, I don't know what else I would like to do, or could do."

"Anyway" he continued, "I've got you in here because I thought you might like to see a little procedure I need to do from time to time."

Striding out into the ward, he went to where Norman sat in his wheelchair and proceeded to wheel him into the clinic, and then closed the door behind him. Norman was a very quite and unassuming man of around seventy, whose wheelchair was always parked in the same place close by the office. Apparently he had a shrapnel wound in his leg while serving in the army, during the war. The wound would, every so often, need draining off as fluid built up inside it, making his leg swell up as a result. I haven't much recollection of how Henry carried out the 'operation,' but I remember feeling partly revolted by it, yet feeling very pleased that I was able to witness it. Afterwards I wheeled Norman back onto the ward again, by which time the shift was nearly over.

"Come with me will you Robert." Frank called over to me as he emerged from the office, while I was putting the breaks on the wheelchair.

He was carrying a torch as we entered the dormitory, which by now was very quiet with the only light being from the nightlight situated near to the doorway of the dayroom. He spoke softly as he explained that every patient had to be counted both at the beginning of the shift and again at the end, before the ward was handed over to the next shift.

Typically Frank, always did the last count himself when on duty, and it wasn't just a head count either. As he moved from one bed to another checking each patient was breathing and being careful not to shine the torch directly into his face, he adjusted a sheet, or a pillow as he thought necessary, so as to make each patient comfortable.

Over the next few nights while we were on the late shift, Frank would always ask me to accompany him in this duty. Now, I know that it may sound silly, but I enjoyed that more than anything else I remember from my early days of nursing. I felt like a male version of Florence nightingale and for those few moments of the shift I couldn't think of anywhere else I would rather be in the world. It made all the other things that we had to do worthwhile; things such as dealing with uncooperative patients who wanted to do one thing while we were desperately trying to get them to do another, this and the many other frustrations involved in each shift seemed to pale into insignificance as I walked slowly around the ward at night with Frank.

That night I was again allowed to go home early, only by about ten minutes, but as I put my own key into the door to let myself out I felt so much better about things, not happy exactly, but much happier.

Chapter 5

For the rest of that two weeks I really knuckled down to working on the ward, partly to prove to myself that I was capable and also because I wanted Frank to approve of me.

If there was a patient that needed changing due to incontinence, or if there was someone that wanted toileting, I'd be there instantly. The most enthusiastic member of the team, I learnt all the patient's names and I waited to intervene at any moment, should there be a need. There were a number of them that were unsteady on their feet and if they started to wander I would fetch one of the restraining chairs, should it become necessary. Years later these same chairs became outlawed, but then, if anyone persisted in wandering around and were in danger of falling and hurting themselves these chairs were to be used as the method of containing them.

I tried to talk to the patients to find out what they did for a living, trying to see in those who seemed to have a recollection of the past if there were things that I could resurrect. What I found with some was that they might have been disoriented as to the time and the place that they were in at present, but they were often able to give an account of things that were long gone.

It was during this time I gave my first injection. Traditionally the 'first time' was done using an orange, but as luck would have it there was a patient who was suffering from a chest infection and needed an injection, and I was there, and so was Maurice.

"I shouldn't really be letting you do this," Maurice whispered as we sat next to the patient in the dormitory, "but I thought you'd want to, so I'll let you do this jab."

I was only too pleased. I was also very nervous, but wanted to get as much experience under my belt as possible before I started my training. The injection was to be in the patient's buttock.

Well, I did it, I can't remember now how it felt, but I was pleased to have done something so 'nursey.'

Back to the patients, because if it weren't for them there wouldn't be anything to write about, nor would there have been any psychiatric hospitals.

Ben was my favourite, although professionally speaking there should never be a favourite of course, but I couldn't help myself, every spare moment I had I sat with them all and tried to talk with them, especially Ben. He was about eighty years old, bent almost double when he walked, leaning heavily on a stick and supported on the other side by a nurse. He had a huge scrotal hernia, probably due to hard work as a farm labourer. It was big, very big, and some of the staff used to refer to it as a cannon ball, when they saw it exposed while giving him a bath. I suppose that I ought to have spoken out, but being a newcomer I didn't really feel that I could, yet inside I felt really sorry that they could joke with him about such a thing.

Looking back now I wish I could undo some of the wrongs that, although were probably meant in all innocence, were unkind as well as unprofessional, not only on Devon ward, but throughout those early years. I should have told the unfeeling nurses who said such things to have some empathy, some pity, and some professionalism. Sadly I remained silent, to my eternal shame.

Fortunately the nurses who ill-treated the patients either mentally, or physically were few and far between.

In those days patients had few rights and in all walks of life there's always the odd rotten apple in the barrel. Harry didn't say a lot, but I'm sure that he felt it when he was the butt of their jokes. Although he didn't speak much at any time, he did remember his days on the farm as a child and as an adult and he seemed to make sense when he spoke. I don't remember much of it, only that he had a very dry sense of humour and if he was in a certain frame of mind he would sit and talk and make me really laugh.

The only thing though was that, with his stick he'd rake up anything that he saw lying on the floor, and reaching down, he'd take it between two fingers, place it in his mouth and chew it. Fine if it was a cigarette end, but sometimes it might be, and sometimes was a small piece of faeces!

I also rather liked Ralph, who could be difficult if he felt like it, yet everyone liked him. At various times during the day cigarettes were given to those who wanted them, Ralph was one of those who wanted a smoke. The only thing is that if he wasn't first in line for one he'd get up from his seat and begin to shout out,

"Ain't got none. Ain't got none. Give it me, give it me."

If he didn't get one immediately he'd let out the most horrific roar, or rather, roars! In the meantime he would descend on whoever was nearest to him with a cigarette and attempt to wrestle it from their hand. It could be quite scary, but I'm pretty sure in my own mind that some of the staff kept his cigarette until last just for the entertainment value. Funnily enough Ralph never normally spoke very much unless he was agitated about something.

Reg was another patient on the ward. Nobody liked him except Norman the man with the shrapnel wound. The staff and patients tried to avoid him if at all possible, for good reason. Reg had been a farmer, quite a wealthy one, but at some time or another he had been kicked by his prize bull and now only walked with the aid of a walking frame. He was moody and aggressive in his manner and if one of the patients annoyed him he would lash out and try and either hit him, or trip him up. He was very rude and ungrateful and altogether quite an unpleasant man and I didn't believe that he was particularly mentally ill, just rather nasty. However for some reason Norman and Reg got on really well and they would sit next to each other all day without a bad word between them.

One evening towards the end of the week I met Nigel, who was one of the regular night nurses, and Henry's ex partner. He was an SEN. and was not only gay, but also one of the funniest men that I'd met up until that point. All the staff loved him, especially the females. I can't for the life of me remember a single conversation with him, which is rather sad, and I never had the chance to work with him. Whenever I had the opportunity I sought out his company, as many others did, just to listen to his fantastic humour.

I once recall his scathing remark in reply to a female nurse, who told him she had bought some beauty product,

"You don't want to buy that rubbish, dear," he retorted. "Buy some decent stuff, like this!" he flicked out his hand so that she could have a smell of his wrist.

He adored Mae West one of the old Hollywood stars and loved to imitate her.

His "Come up and see me sometime," and

"When I'm good, I'm good and when I'm bad I'm better," was to me as near to the original as you could get.

Along with his excellent sense of humour and quick wit, he was a brilliant nurse, too. Frank thought that he was great and whenever he was on duty overnight he knew that his patients were going to get five star treatment.

Unfortunately this wasn't always the case in nursing, especially with night nurses. Later on in my career hopefully I became a good one myself, but often they weren't up to the mark, they just wanted to do the minimum amount of work and put their feet up for a snooze! But not everyone was like that and Nigel was a good example of the caring night nurse. He made sure, that every one of the patients were washed and that all their needs were fully met and more besides. Unfortunately his own mother became infirm and within a few months of my being there he left us to look after her.

It's always seemed strange to me why many gay men are so close to their mothers and Nigel was an example of this. Over the years I've worked with many gay people, men in particular, and I've always been impressed at how caring many of them are, and how meticulous in their duties. Before arriving at the hospital I don't think that I'd come across any gay men, or women, but working with them in nursing I've really appreciated their dedication to their patients and have very much enjoyed their marvellous sense of humour as a general rule.

The Friday night of that first week was the end of my duties for a couple of days. Because of the way the rota ran it was my weekend off. I was relieved to have some time to myself as, working afternoons made the mornings useless, there didn't seem to be time to do anything before I was due to go on duty.

I can't remember how I spent the weekend, but I know that I found it was very difficult to get out of bed at six o clock in the morning on the following Monday to get ready for work. I never got into the habit of getting up early; it always remained a problem to me. It reminded me of when I used to work on the bread deliveries, having to be at the depot halfway through the night. In summer it wasn't too bad, walking through the arboretum at the break of day it was a joy to hear the sound of the dawn chorus. But as I made my way to work in the winter it was a different story, I hated the cold and the rain and just wanted to stay nice and warm in my bed.

However I arrived on time for this first morning shift at seven o clock, not knowing what lay ahead. I'd only worked afternoon shifts on Devon ward.

It was awful; if I thought that the afternoon shift was hard work this was torture.

Firstly there was a welcome cup of tea. That was all right. Then came the handover. Henry would come, or if he was off duty the senior nurse would come and tell us anything that was relevant for the shift. After that it was all systems go.

Most of the patients were still in bed and needed to be got up for breakfast. We worked like crazy, in teams of two. Many of the patients were wet and needed washing and shaving before being dressed.

Some were covered in faeces, having been incontinent before we reached them. If you've never dealt with a doubly incontinent patient who is agitated and is smearing it all over the place, well, you certainly don't want to experience it! Some of them would have 'it' on their hands and even their faces, certainly on other parts of their bodies. We called it being tished up.

Well, I plunged in, so to speak, and sometimes was lucky and I and the other nurse managed to get the patient to the breakfast table without any real problems, but other times it was a nightmare! It wasn't just that they were soiled; the worst thing is that they resisted everything that we were trying to do for them. One of us had to hold the patients hands; the other had to do the honours. It seems a bit callous, but at the end of the day we had a job to do and a deadline for breakfast.

If the patients weren't on time, Lorna just would not wait; she would take the trolley away with the breakfast in it. Mind you the patients who didn't get there on time still had their breakfast, it just meant that one of the nursing staff had to go to the kitchen and put several breakfasts onto plates and put them in the oven for when the patients were ready.

I found over the next few years that many of the ward orderlies and cleaners were difficult, they seemed to like their bit of power, not having an understanding of mental illness. They'd sometimes be off hand and rude to the patients, and regarded the kitchen as their very own domain, only allowing entry to those they approved of. I suppose in fairness they were right, as there were hot plates and knives, as well as other potentially dangerous instruments, so a confused patient could harm himself, or someone else.

Apart from that though, some of them were very bossy, shouting at an unsuspecting person who walked on their newly polished floor, or giving the evil eye to another who had done some minor sin in their eyes. They seemed to want as little to do with the patients as possible, except to scold them, which seemed to me ridiculous, as the patients were what the hospital was all about.

Not all domestics were like that of course, some were very kind to the patients, getting them to help with chores such as laying the tables, not because they were lazy themselves, but because they were genuinely fond of them. Also they knew that while the patients were busily employed doing something like that, nursing staff were given a bit of a hand, and it was occupational therapy for the patient.

On some of the wards the domestics worked with the nurses as a part of the team. Occasionally, they would sneak an extra cup of tea to one or two of the patients, and sometimes sat talking to them. Others even brought little treats in, to say ‘thank you’ if one or another had helped out with the washing up, or cleaning.

Unfortunately there were lazy ones; some wards weren’t as clean as they might have been, and in spite of the domestic supervisor coming around frequently, to check on them they still sloped off for numerous cigarettes during their shift. Mind you I knew of at least one who because he had upset the charge nurse was taken off the wards and given the endless job of washing and polishing the hospital corridors and there must have been miles of them; I think he left a short time afterwards.

After breakfast and medication it was time for another cup of tea for the staff. Officially we were allowed only one tea break per shift, but in reality we often squeezed an extra one in. Even most of the nursing officers would turn a blind eye to this practice, some of them occasionally joining us for a while if they were passing through. Personally I didn’t enjoy their company, as the conversation would often become stilted when they sat at the table with us, and I usually felt quiet threatened by their company, a feeling that stayed with me for the whole of my career, I always seemed to find the presence of seniors uncomfortable.

Following the tea break there were beds to make and patients to be bathed; on this ward it was usually a morning job. We were split into three teams, one team kept an eye on the patients in the day room, another went to do bed making, and the other was destined for the bathroom. I can't recall making any beds in that first couple of weeks, but I clearly recall the bathing!

First of all we didn't have any hoists in the bathrooms in those days, or if they were available on a few of the wards they weren't often used. The method we used follows.

First go and find a poor unsuspecting victim encourage him to come to the bathroom, and to undress, or be undressed, though sometimes unwillingly. During which time the nurse who wasn't doing the undressing was filling the bath, cold-water tap first of course. The patient, if he could stand was then assisted into the bath, if he couldn't he was bodily lifted into the tub, and then a jug of water was poured over the patient's head. If the nurse was kind he, or she would attempt to prevent the water going into the eyes, but that wasn't always the case.

After the patient had been thoroughly washed, he was assisted out of the bath. Easy enough if he happened to be mobile, but if not a bath towel was used, ensuring that there was a chair situated at the end of the bath, The towel was threaded under the arms with the ends sticking out towards the front of the patient, then both nurses would get either side of him, take one end of the towel each and pull. If they pulled heartily enough the patient would end up on the chair at the end of the bath, if not then he would sink down into the water again and we would have to try again.

It may seem a bit primitive, but at the time it was the only way that we knew how to do the task. This bad practice was passed down the line, each new student doing the same thing.

Now things are very different, but it took a long while for things to change, as people dislike any changes, especially if things are done too quickly. When hoists were introduced as standard to the wards which, was a long way into my career, many of the older nurses didn't want to use them, because they were too complicated, and to them, unnecessary. There were many training sessions before they became truly accepted.

There were other things, of course that had to be done, especially as the patients were highly dependant on the nursing staff to meet their needs.

For instance there were dressings to be seen to on various types of wounds, usually leg ulcers associated with diabetes, or there were pressure areas that needed attending to, due to many of the patients sitting for long periods on totally unsuitable chairs. But for me, my time on the morning shift was spent mostly in getting the patients up, feeding them and then bathing them. By the time that was all over it was time for a quick break and perhaps afterwards supervising several patients with their cigarettes, trying to ensure that those who did smoke didn't get them taken from them by the more unscrupulous and desperate patients who wanted more than one; and then it was lunch.

This routine went on for the rest of the week with Frank occasionally intervening to show me either a simple procedure that he thought I might benefit from, or allowing me into the office for a while so that I might look at the patients dossiers, in order that I could find out a little more of the patients histories.

I don't recall, if I'm honest what the dossiers contained, only that some of the patients had been there since the nineteen thirties, and more than one longer than that. I looked through their histories and found that several had, in the early days of their admission, been extremely violent at times.

Of course in those days they didn't have the modern medicines that we have now, and I wondered how on earth the staff had coped. Not only that but they were sometimes admitted for the most trivial of reasons, for instance causing a disturbance in the neighbourhood, and instead of spending just a few weeks in the hospital for assessment, they seemed to have been incarcerated for life. I found out later that was particularly true also for those who were unmarried mothers, particularly if they had had the baby taken away from them and had become distressed as a result, and had perhaps slid down into a depression.

Thankfully Friday lunchtime saw my last shift on the ward and although I was happy to have had the experience and believed that it would stand me in good stead for the next six weeks in nursing school, I was glad when One-Fifteen p.m. on Friday came and I could go home. I had escaped another weekend, because on the Monday I was to start my journey as a student nurse, I wondered what it would be like. Surely it had to be better than the last two weeks. I thanked Frank and the rest of the staff hoping that I wouldn't see them again in the near future, and then closing the door behind me I beat a hasty retreat.

Chapter 6.

On Monday morning I made my way to the training school, which was attached to the nurses accommodation block. I was nervous, but felt that the last two weeks on Devon ward had given me an advantage over what I thought would be a load of raw recruits in my PTS. I was soon to be enlightened in that area! On arriving I sat in the classroom listening to the various conversations going on while we waited for the tutor to arrive. It seemed that out of sixteen of us most of the group knew each other and had been at St. Andrews for a great deal longer than myself. I suddenly felt very alone and vulnerable.

After a few minutes Rees came into the room.

"I think that nearly all of you know me," he said, "but for those who don't, my name is Rees Jones, I will be your main tutor for the next six weeks."

He went on to say that we could call him Rees, but that as a matter of respect, unless invited to call any other tutor by their first name we must use their surname, as most of those that would be lecturing would be nursing officer grade.

The next thing on the agenda was to introduce ourselves in turn, telling the rest of the class something about our past lives and what we had done before we took up nursing, also we were encouraged to share our previous experience if any, in nursing. Well, I was really feeling inferior after that! Many of the group, which consisted mainly of young people, with only two of them older than myself, had either entered nursing as cadets at the age of sixteen, or had a parent who was working as a nurse. Others had worked as HCA's for several years before deciding to do their training. Only three, I think had no previous knowledge of working in a hospital and they were foreign students.

When this session was over we were told that we could get ourselves a cup of tea, or coffee in a room adjoining the classroom. As we stood and drank we talked among ourselves and I started to relax a little as we began to mingle and to get to know one another. There was one lad, I conversed with who had a motorbike, which was the love of his life, and he told me

"It only does as many miles to the gallon as the average car, but it really goes. The thing is, you can overtake anything, and I bet you if I am trying to get to the same place as you, I'll get there first."

I tried to sound impressed, but to me it seemed all so ridiculous. I couldn't understand how anyone would want to ride around in the open, getting freezing cold when they could be all cosy in a car, and to put the same amount of petrol in his tank as well, seemed stupidity. I didn't tell him that of course, well not on the first day, anyway.

Fiona, a young girl who had been a cadet and had always wanted to be a nurse came from a family of nurses, all of whom worked at St. Andrews. I would later be staffed on the same ward as her dad, an amiable Irishman and a charge nurse, who, I'm afraid taught me nothing except how to while away the shift talking about the old days in Ireland.

Raj, was an Indian Mauritian, who I discovered later on made the most beautiful curry. I was only ever to taste this delight once, but the experience will never fade from my memory, my mouth waters as I write!

Of course eventually I got to know all of them, but before long our first tea break was over and we were called back to the classroom. There, Rees gave us a brief history of nursing and of how it had developed. If I remember rightly, Bethlehem Royal Hospital, known, as Bedlam was the first mental hospital in the country, although it was then known as an asylum. The patients were referred to as idiots, or lunatics, and he told us, if we looked back into some of the dossiers of those of our older patients that had been in the hospital for most of their lives we would perhaps find examples of such terminology.

In the nineteenth century, before the advent of medication, one of the treatments that was popular with disturbed patients was to give them hot and cold baths, alternately. Straight jackets, of course were used as a means of restraint, also padded cells. St. Andrews still had a few of these on some of the wards. They weren't used in our day, naturally, and were all ripped out by the time I had moved on, but all of these things were part of the past.

There is an understanding nowadays of the importance of the relationship between the nurse and his or her patient. Tranquillisers, anti depressants and all the other medication were helpful, of course and necessary, but the nurse/patient relationship was an essential part of the management of someone with a mental illness.

It seems strange to me now, that we were taught that all those years ago and yet there is so much more paperwork nowadays than there was then and as a result the trained psychiatric nurses appear to be so weighed down with it all, that most of their time is spent in the office dealing with it instead of being out on the ward with their patients. The HCA's are the ones that spend the majority of the shift with the patients.

Anyway, then it was time for lunch, so off we sauntered to the staff canteen to sample the subsidised food, and very tasty it was too. I know that some people aren't keen on hospital food, but I for one liked it; mind you I liked school dinners as well, I don't suppose that says very much for my dear mums cooking. These breaks were an ideal time to get to know each other and enjoy a bit of banter together.

That first day it was alright, things in the classroom weren't too heavy, but as we got further and further into the course we found that these times together were good for clearing our heads, and on my part at least, to prevent me from descending into a deep depression as I realised how miserably unlearned I was. It wasn't that I didn't know much, after all that was what the lectures were all about, they were to teach us; with me it was something more fundamental.

As the weeks progressed and we got into anatomy and physiology and all the other things that we were required to know, I found myself struggling. Why hadn't I spent more time listening to the teachers at school, instead of messing about? If I struggled in those early lectures it was even worse when a little later we began to delve into the nervous, and vascular systems and then a little psychology, not forgetting the endocrine system, the different types of schizophrenia, the signs and symptoms of various illnesses, etc, etc. I always felt out of my depth, always interrupting the lecturer to ask 'just one more question.'

In fact I think that there was only one other person in the class that was as lost as me, poor old Eddie, he was a big teddy bear of a lad in his late teens, he had been a nursing cadet and had that advantage. Apparently he had been a hard worker on the wards and was well liked by patients and staff alike, but like me, when it came to the classroom he couldn't really handle it.

After a year of training we were obliged to take an intermediate exam. Eddie failed, but he was allowed time to do some more studying and to try again, but again he failed. We felt so very sorry for him, especially as he was the only one who was not allowed to continue his training. Eddie went back onto the wards again for a time, but I suppose the humiliation of having to work with some of us as we continued our training must have pushed him into resigning. What a pity, just because he wasn't academic didn't make him a bad nurse.

As the six weeks progressed it wasn't all doom and gloom, there were lighter moments too. Such as the time when during a break I took the skeleton out of the cupboard where it hung, and placed it on a chair at the side of me, much to the amusement of the rest of the students. Miss Boyde came in a few minutes later and there was, naturally a lot of sniggering going on, she called us to order and commenced her lecture and completed it without so much of a glance in the skeletons direction. I have to say this about Miss Boyde, she was our least favourite tutor, not only did she seem devoid of a sense of humour, but also she didn't appreciate it if we asked questions during her lectures.

Rumour had it that she had recently left her husband of many years and had set up home with a female social worker that worked in the hospital. Due to this I was always curious about her. To me, naïve as I was and having, I imagine led rather a sheltered life I couldn't quite figure out why she would want to do such a thing, and call herself 'Miss' to boot.

During the rest of my time as a student I got to know Miss Boyde quite well and found her to be quite a nice person outside of the school. She helped me tremendously with my practical assessments, which were a requirement of the course.

One day I plucked up the courage to ask her if she had noticed the skeleton.

"Of course, but it was rather boring, nearly every PTS. does the same thing," she answered dryly. That knocked me off of my perch!

I suppose I may as well share something else. When as an innocent applicant for nurse training I was considering the type of people who would be part of the caring profession, I thought back to my younger sisters books that I used to pick up and read from time to time, as a child. The nurses in the books always seemed as if they were almost heavenly beings, angelic in their appearance, and in the performance of their duties.

When as an eight year old lad I had to spend a week in hospital for something quite minor, I distinctly remember falling head over heels in love with one of the nurses, who was to me, indeed like an angel. At the end of my stay I was reluctantly dragged from the ward having been discharged and taken back home. On my arrival there, before many minutes had gone by I crept out of the house and ran to the public toilets halfway down our street, locking myself in one of the lavatories, I burst into uncontrollable sobbing and a little later, when it was out of my system I walked back home feeling totally miserable; I had lost my angel!

During these first few weeks training as a nurse myself, I found things to be utterly different from what I had expected. Not that I'm making judgements, just reflecting and explaining how things appeared to me at that time.

For instance Frank, whom I greatly admired was living with what we today would call a partner. Henry was homosexual, Nigel too. Kat, I had been told was having an affair with Maurice and she was a married woman with children.

This was all within a couple of weeks of my starting nursing, what would I learn about later on? Later I found that the hospital was rife with affairs and broken marriages. Later on my own half brother lost his wife because she was then working at St. Andrews and had an affair with a male nurse, whom I knew and had never really liked even before I found out about their indiscretion.

I know that all this sounds as though I'm being terribly judgemental, but I'm not really. I came from a family that knew what it was to be in the middle of a marriage breakdown, as my own father left home when I was twelve years old. Oh, so shameful at the time. Free school dinners, free school uniforms purchased using a voucher. The neighbours comments, and I'm not just talking about the adults, I'm referring to the children I went to school with, not to mention my aunties and my grandmother calling round to bring my sisters and I somebody else's cast offs. And also the snidey remarks made by my grandma about my mum, whom she'd never really liked, even though grandma had never got on with my dad, (her son) anyway.

I just didn't expect it to be like this at the hospital. I expected Florence Nightingale type characters, but on top of this, later in my training I came across those who were supposed to be caring, only to find them sometimes uncaring. Not all of them, of course by any means, but the ones who were less than perfect in this respect tarnished the dream I had of nurses being akin to angels.

After a while I awakened from my dream and faced reality, there were no angels in nursing, only ordinary people, some good and some not so good. Over the years I did meet a great many who were, if not angelic, at least rather saintly.

I've never met Mother Theresa, but I've met a number of nurses who would have been worthy of working alongside of her. Mind you I don't really know why I should have expected to see any heavenly beings, as upon reflection I was no angel myself!

During those weeks our PTS. group began to knit together. Several of the students began to date and in fact two couples eventually married, (though one couple divorced shortly afterwards, due to an affair with another nurse.) Another couple began to live together and as far as I know they are still together.

I discovered that one of the others, Tim had been a motor mechanic before he had entered nursing. What a blessing that was to me and to some of the others later on, as problems cropped up with our cars. Our wages could barely feed us, let alone pay for repair bills for our motors, but good old Tim helped us out whenever he could, often spending a whole precious day off duty to fix things for us. Another thing that involved money was that we were required to buy certain books, which was going to be expensive, except that we came upon the idea of sharing. Instead of buying all the books ourselves, we each bought one or two and passed them around in a sort of a rota system.

I was befriended by one of the older students named Maggie; she wasn't really old, just old compared with the rest of us. She very kindly used to bring in home made cakes for me, as she learned that I had a sweet tooth.

Stephen, another a member of our group would share the travelling expenses to and from the hospital with me, by sometimes using his car, sometimes mine, during those six weeks in school and in fact for some time afterwards. Mind you there was an interlude of a few weeks when Stephen left his wife and moved in with Sally, a very attractive and vivacious member of our group. Stephens wife had an alcohol problem and he also suspected that she was having an affair, so he left her for Sally, but it didn't last very long and he eventually moved back in with his wife, more for his little boys sake than anything else, I think.

On one occasion when one of the group wanted to get away early for some reason one afternoon, we put the clock forward and the tutor let us go before our time. Mind you we got a strip torn off us the next day when he realised he'd been duped.

Apart from the serious side of learning there was a lot of good fun, like the time I did my Elvis Presley imitation to rapturous applause. Little did I know that shortly afterwards Elvis would be dead!

Bella, a coloured nurse from Nigeria one day stuck a pillow under her jumper and ran around the room calling out,

"Look, I'm pregnant, I don't know how it happened!"

"You've done gone been a bad girl!" I cried out in my best deep southern state, black American voice. The classroom was in uproar, the tutor, of course wasn't present.

Naturally, today I couldn't make such a joke as I would probably be accused of being racist, but in those days it was accepted for what it was; just a bit of fun.

Life in PTS. wasn't all fun, much of the time we worked hard; in fact there was an awful lot of hard work. I filled several exercise books up with my note taking, as I'm sure the others did.

We were taught that to be a nurse one must respect confidentiality, but be prepared to report anything that a patient told us if it was deemed important, and not to enter into any secrecy pact with the patient, agreeing to withhold something that might be relevant to their well being. We were to be non judgemental. "There, but for the grace of God go I." Rees told us with conviction.

"Everyone must be treated with respect, regardless of his, or her mental state."

I learned the difference between sympathy and empathy; not only feeling for the patient but being able, if possible to put ourselves in their place and indeed, how awful it must have been to have been admitted to a mental hospital. Not only to feel ill and confused, but to be surrounded by others who were in the same situation, yet all exhibiting their own different symptoms and behaviour; it must have seemed like hell on earth to have that thrust upon anyone who was unfortunate enough to experience it.

We were told that no one is ‘normal,’ all having traits that might be thought of as a part of a mental illness. For example there are a good many people who are fanatical about keeping their car clean, they could be thought of as obsessional. Others might worry about every day things such as whether they have enough money to live on, when in fact they earn a very good wage. These people could be thought of as having a form of neurosis. Silly examples, I know, but I think you get the gist. Then came the lesson on how to make a bed with Hospital corners of course, starting with the bottom sheet at the head of the bed, not at the bottom of the bed, which inevitably was my mistake.

Afterwards Sally showed us how to make an apple pie bed, which was, to the untrained eye a normally made up bed, but in fact the sheets had been folded in such a way that it was impossible to get into it.

First aid was also among the delights that we learned, with everyone getting the bandages and slings on the wrong way round, at least at the first attempt.

All of us had to have a go at reviving the dummy, on which we learned resuscitation, we called her by a name which I’ve forgotten after all this time. Of course some of the brighter sparks in the group had tried to have a passionate kiss with her, for once, I wasn't among those sad individuals!

There were also practical procedures to be learned such as bed baths and how to use a bedpan. If you think that's easy you ought to try it sometime, I never did get the hang of it properly.

During some of the lectures we were shown a selection of the bottles that were filled with pickled organs, some of which graced the shelves and windowsills of the classroom. The type of organ was revealed to us as the lecture progressed, and we naturally had them on view during the anatomy and physiology lectures for reference purposes, much to my and several other of the group's disgust, apparently some of them were extremely old.

We were at some time during our PTS. shown around a few of the wards by Mrs. Halloway the wife of the senior tutor. She was a friendly woman in her mid forties who was soon to leave her husband for what reason I don't know, it just seemed to be the norm at St. Andrews for marriages to break down.

The first ward that she took us to was a large house that stood apart from the main building and was filled with women who mostly seemed to be middle aged and who I would later come to know as 'characters,' not those patients in particular of course, but many of the long stay patients in the hospital. A girl in our group, obviously being familiar with one of the patients spoke to her in order to get some sort of reaction and was told bluntly by Mrs. Halloway not to bait the patients.

We moved on from there and saw inside several of the wards, but all of them were long stay, not acute wards which I was the most interested in, having come into nursing to deal specifically with that type of patient; again I was disappointed.

A few days before the end of the six-week session I was called into the office by Rees, who asked me, that in view of all the questions I had been plying the tutors with during their lectures, if I felt that I was cut out for nursing. He was concerned that I might perhaps have overstretched myself, and wanted to reassure himself that I would be able to complete the three-year course successfully.

I was devastated, and embarrassed by this and insisted that I did want to go on and that I was sure that I would make it, and rambling on, I told him that the only reason that I asked so many questions was that I wanted to clarify everything, 'Not just for myself,' I lied, 'but for all of the group.' He seemed satisfied with this and let me go.

As I left for home that night though, I felt humiliated and useless. How could I face them all again?

Still I did, turning up the next morning as if nothing had happened. I was quiet of course, not asking any questions, the rest noticed and remarked, but I didn't tell them what had happened, and I kept a low profile for the rest of the time that was left of the six weeks.

The end of the PTS. exam came upon us quickly. None of us were looking forward to it even the brightest of the stars among us, but it was inevitable. Stephen came around to my house for several nights in a row beforehand and we revised all the information that had been fed into us over the weeks.

During every tea and lunch breaks for a few days before the dreaded test I went through my note books like a man possessed, and on the morning of the exam I was feeling numb with all the studying. Still it seemed to go all right, and we all went down to the notice board afterwards as requested, to find out where our first ward placement would be. We all hoped for an acute admission ward, of course, because they were the most coveted placements. What did I get? Devon ward! Of all the wards! At least, if I had to get a sick ward it wouldn't have hurt to have been placed on another, so that I could get a wider variety of experience, but no, for me it was Devon.

I discovered later, after complaining to Rees, that Frank had asked for me especially because he believed that I would benefit from three months under his wing. Three months was the length of each placement and I wasn't looking forward to it, in fact I was downright resentful. Most of the others in the group tripped off merrily to spend a well-earned weekend away from all the studying and looking forward to their next twelve weeks; I trudged slowly towards my car feeling cheated.

In a couple of weeks time I found out that I had passed the exam, but with a miserable score of around sixty six percent, most of the others had managed to get into the seventies, or even eighties. After each session in the classroom we had to sit a test and I was always down the bottom of the class, why was I being so dense? I found it all so very embarrassing, especially as I seemed to spend much more time studying than the rest, yet I still wasn't getting the results; it was all so depressing.

I never went out with the others on their drinking sessions or socialised in the staff club, like the rest of the PTS. I wanted to get home to my family and whenever possible spend time at the church meetings, which was becoming more difficult now because of the shift system. I felt that it was worth it though, but if only I could do better in the classroom.

Chapter 7.

The resentment I felt at being placed back on Devon ward didn't last long, because when on Monday afternoon I arrived on the ward I was greeted by familiar faces who seemed genuinely pleased to see me and kept on calling me student nurse.

"Student nurse Panton," Kat would call out for no particular reason, pretending that she needed a hand with something, then laughing her socks off as I hurried to help her. Of course I couldn't run now, that wasn't allowed as a student, or ever afterward, only in any real emergency.

The ward was still as I remembered it, with Ralph, as usual bawling out

"I ain't got none," while the cigarettes were being handed around to the patients.

Before long Billy was shouting,

"I'm wet, wet, wet, wet, wet."

I know that you may think that I am making it up to make things sound more interesting, but that really is exactly as I remember it. Maurice who was still on the ward went to pacify Ralph, giving him the much needed cigarette, then putting an affectionate arm around him, he only had it shrugged off, to make it easier for him to smoke the longed for and coveted treasure, the cigarette, then someone went to rescue Billy.

Naturally, before too many minutes had passed there was the inevitable toilet round with Wilf calling out

"Aye. Aye," as I took him to the lavatory. All was as normal, just the way I'd left it six weeks before, and funnily enough it was ok.

In a strange way I felt at home. I didn't want to be there, yet somehow I didn't want to be anywhere else.

During the tea break Frank came to the table and sat down for a quick cup of tea. On leaving the table he asked me to follow him into the dormitory. Before we went through the door he spoke in a low voice to me.

"We have a new admission from one of the other wards. It isn't very good, I'm afraid and we'll need to give an awful lot of input if this man is to survive."

By his tone I realised that he was worried and I followed him in silence. Sam lay on a bed in the middle of the right hand side of the dormitory; he had been sent to us about a week before and had deteriorated severely in the past couple of days. When we approached his eyes were closed, he appeared to be around about seventy years old and quite thin.

"He's emaciated and dehydrated," Frank whispered.

"But worse, look at this!"

As he spoke he pulled the bedcovers down, revealing Sam's sacral area, he had a large dressing on each side.

"We need to get on top of before it gets any worse," he said softly, always aware that the patient might be listening and maybe become distressed as a result of our conversation.

Frank went to wash his hands, after wheeling a trolley loaded with dressings and instruments to the side of the bed. He got me to roll Sam onto one side; he then removed the dressing and using a swab, poured some solution onto a black area of the bedsore. The solution caused a sort of fizzing, and then he used another swab to clean around the cavity that was surrounding the necrotic area. Finally he cleansed the skin that was intact and he then packed the cavity with a saline dressing. The same procedure was repeated on the other side. The smell was disgusting, unlike anything that I had smelt before enough to make me recoil from it instinctively, enough certainly to make one vomit, except I knew that I had to be strong!

Sadly it wasn't the last time that I encountered such a vile smell. Sam groaned at times during the procedure, but was too weak to put up any resistance, which, at least made the job a lot easier and quicker than it might have been.

After Frank had finished placing a dressing over each wound we laid Sam on his back and propped him up with pillows before leaving him.

When we were back in the office Frank told me that Sam had come in from one of the long stay wards, who weren't able to cope with him anymore due to the high level of physical care that was now needed. It was now time for the sick ward to intervene.

"But, why did they leave it so long?" I asked, concerned that he had been allowed to get into such a state.

"I don't know," Frank replied, "All I do know is that here and there you'll find as you progress in your nursing career, some of the care isn't what it should be. This patient has been in bed without anyone giving attention to his skin care. Anyone who is in bed for any length of time needs to be, at the very least turned regularly, if they can't do it for themselves. This man hasn't been looked after properly, and I want you to remember him and any others that you come across who seem to have been neglected, as you continue your training, so that in the future when you eventually have charge of a ward, this sort of thing doesn't happen."

I nodded in agreement, feeling sad about Sam, but also quite flattered that Frank thought that one day I might have my own ward.

The rest of the shift went as normal except that I was asked to feed Sam some fluids during the early evening. Using a feeder cup. I made some headway and was able to record on the sheet at the bottom of his bed that I'd given him a cup of orange juice although I had to admit that he coughed and spluttered over it. As we did the normal check of the patients that night Frank was far from satisfied.

"If things are no better tomorrow and if the morning staff haven't done it, I think I will insert a naso gastric tube," he said, looking concerned.

That night I went home thinking about the situation and finding myself so upset that I didn't get to sleep until the early hours. This would be the normal thing for me, on and off for the rest of my career. It was sometimes impossible to switch off, especially if there was someone that you were concerned about on your ward.

The next afternoon I was spared the toileting routine as Frank asked me to help him. On the one hand I felt guilty and thought that the other staff would be resentful, but on the other hand I was relieved, not to say intrigued as to what was to happen next.

Apparently the morning staff had tried without success to feed Sam, so Frank had called the doctor over, he was there when I entered the dormitory. Frank already had a trolley by the bed and drew the curtains round as I approached, beckoning me in to watch. A tube was inserted into the patients nose and passed down into the stomach so liquid nutrition could be given. When the doctor was quite sure that it was in the right place he taped the remainder of the tube to Sams face and left the ward.

It was the staffs job to take it in turns every couple of hours syringing fluids into the tube in an effort to re-hydrate him, I'm not sure, on reflection why a drip wasn't used, but all I know is that it was several years before I ever saw anyone on a drip in St. Andrews, usually patients needing that sort of intervention were sent to the general hospital.

Anyway Sam benefited from a great deal of personal care over the next several days. His dressings were done daily and his pressure areas attended to, as well as us constantly giving him fluids. Sadly he became less and less responsive and on the Friday evening he died.

I was there for his last few moments and went to call for Frank, as he reached the bedside I asked

"Is he gone?"

Frank held a finger up to his mouth and then checked in vain for signs of life. After he had satisfied himself that Sam had indeed died, he drew me to one side, while another nurse opened a window, to allow the spirit to escape, as was the custom in those days with some of the staff.

Frank explained that the sense of hearing was the last to go when someone dies and that we needed to be careful about what we said at such times.

After about an hour Henry asked me to do the last offices with him. I'll not go through the procedure, suffice it to say that even though things are done somewhat differently nowadays, it was done with respect and with a view to the patient's dignity.

Of course Sam's wife was informed, but as she was elderly she didn't want to come out to pay her respects at that moment, so Henry called for the porter and he came with a long metal trolley to take the body away. Sam was taken out of a back door so that the other patients couldn't see, and I assisted the porter with the trolley.

So, after such a short time I had experienced my first death. Not something that I had expected, nor did I suspect that it would have such a deep psychological impact upon me.

I returned home that night as usual, knowing that that weekend I wouldn't have to work.

Fortunately, it had worked out that the rota was in my favour, I say fortunately because for the next two days I was violently sick and felt ghastly. I couldn't help, in my miserable state, but think of Sam. How his body was so cold and grey and still, and eventually, stiff. I couldn't help thinking of how things must have been twenty or thirty years ago. How he and his wife must have laughed together. How perhaps on a Saturday night they may have gone out for a meal together. Perhaps they had grandchildren, and now those little ones had lost the granddad that bounced them on his knee, or chased them around the garden on a summer's afternoon with a water pistol, as they screamed with delight at this loveable old man who was so special to them. And now he was gone; no more the warmth of his body in bed at night, no more the feel of his whiskered face as he kissed the grandchildren goodnight before making his way home with his dear wife.

I thought to myself at that time

'This isn't what I came into nursing for. Let those who want to do it, do it, and I have every admiration for them.' As for me I felt rather like some young lad who had signed up in the army because he thought that it might be a way of learning a trade, only to find that the third world war had started and he was expected to die for his country. I could imagine this young man crying out

"I want my discharge, this isn't how it was meant to be, and I only wanted to play at soldiers, not actually be on the battlefield!"

Life had to go on of course and on Monday morning I presented myself for duty as if nothing had happened. The rest of the staff were, naturally of course on a sick ward, used to death and as far as they were concerned things were back to normal. I never told them, or anyone else for years afterwards, but I was determined to keep death at a respectable distance if I possibly could. Even much later on in my career when I reached the dizzy heights of a charge nurse, although I'd inevitably had the odd brush with death, I would go to any acceptable lengths I could think of to keep the elderly, especially if they were frail, off my ward.

Apart from that, it felt nice to be a part of the team on the ward. Maurice was soon to move on, but the rest would stay and I was now one of them.

One morning I managed to complete a simple crossword in the newspaper that was distributed to every ward, more I suspected for the benefit of the staff than for the patients.

"Are you sure you've done it properly," asked Henry, with a grin. "I knew someone who filled in a crossword, but when he looked at the answers in the next day's paper they were all wrong."

Everybody joined in the fun and ribbed me, as they checked the answers for themselves, even Lorna raised a smile. In fact during that three months Lorna was a lot more amenable towards me, not that she stopped shouting though, if I upset her in some way, but she was much more friendly most of the time. She found it particularly amusing when at Christmas I ate too much Christmas pudding and came onto duty the next day feeling absolutely awful, spending most of the shift in the toilet. I never really liked Christmas pudding after that.

I'd had the Christmas day off, one of the few in my entire nursing career. That was one of the most difficult things I found about being a nurse; while everyone was in their homes with their families, I was on duty pretending to enjoy making all the patient's Christmas jolly, while inside I just wanted to be at home surrounded by my family like most people.

I began to get into the routine after a short while and even found it easier to prepare the patients for bed in the evening. Though there was one incident that makes me shudder even today.

One evening I was getting Matthew into bed when I accidentally trapped his testicles between the bars of one of the cot sides. Matthew had apparently, been a very active member of the Salvation Army and, even though we couldn't get any conversation whatsoever out of him, he did sing a lot of the hymns that he had learned over the years. (The old memories died hard, even if the patients were unable, to tell you what they had for dinner yesterday.) He would also shout out "Hallelujah!" at the top of his voice at intervals during the day, making us all jump out of our skins if we were standing nearby, but I don't think that was the word that he used on that particular occasion.

Another evening Henry was preparing the medicine trolley for the usual round when he dropped a bottle of liquid tranquilliser; there was a mess all over the clinic. It was a sticky substance, which was very difficult to clean up. Hearing the sound of the bottle hitting the floor I was naturally curious, so went to have a look. I laughed so loudly as poor old Henry attempted futilely to sponge it off of his trousers.

"What do you think is so amusing, Panton?" he asked angrily.

Obviously I had underestimated the gravity of the situation, because, before he stormed out of the clinic to find something clean to change into he demanded that I clean up the floor and all the units. What a job that was and how I learned that if something like that happened in the future the best thing was to make oneself scarce!

Another incident that I remember was when one night shortly before we went off duty, I had put the cot sides into position on a particular patients bed. I went to fetch another patient to get him undressed and came back into the dormitory, which had for a short time been left unattended and I saw to my horror that Walter, who I had just left, was standing up on his mattress and was swaying from side to side. Now I know that I wasn't supposed to run, but this was an emergency! Leaving the other patient in his wheelchair I sped towards that bed as fast as I could; but was just too late, he fell over the cot side and landed onto his head. Hearing the noise several other staff members came flying into the dormitory and helped me out; there was blood everywhere. Walter was bundled into a wheelchair, after checking that he was in reasonable order. His wound was cleansed and the duty doctor rushed over to suture the affected area. Fortunately it wasn't as bad as it first appeared and he was later as good as new, if a little bruised. You can guess who was left to clean up all the blood. At least I was given a pair of disposable gloves, which in those days were in short supply.

Another awful thing that happened to me at that time was when one day I was just about to go off duty at lunchtime. Wilf unfortunately had a terrible bout of diarrhoea. I was asked to deal with it because the other staff were busy elsewhere. It wasn't as simple as that though; I took him to the toilet area and removed his trousers and got another pair ready for him, after I had washed him, to my dismay the faeces began to flow again, not only that but he began to use his hands to stem the flow.

My dismay turned to horror.

"Aye. Aye." He repeated over and over again as I tried so hard to take control of the situation.

"Wilf, leave yourself alone, leave it to me," I cried, with more than an element of desperation, because I knew that I should be going off shift an about five minutes

"Aye. Aye." He continued, and at the same time he began wiping his backside with his hands.

After a little while I was absolutely covered in faeces all over the clean white coat that I'd put on that morning.

"Help! Help!" I cried in desperation!

No one came and now in total despair and sweating profusely, I felt absolutely out of my depth, I ran towards the dayroom door and cried out in desperation,

"Will somebody help me out here!"

Then I dashed back to get hold of Wilf before he got the whole of the toilet area covered in the mess.

To my relief one of the afternoon staff came to relieve me, but I was in an awful, smelly state.

The hardest thing that I found about the shift system was working weekends. Of course I had worked them before when I delivered bread, but this was different. Starting at seven o clock, the weekend shift went on until nine at night, with an hour for lunch, it was exhausting!

Naturally as the junior I was expected to participate in the weekend joys of cleaning the sluice, exactly as I'd been warned about. I was also expected to tidy the linen room and the patients clothing room. The latter rooms weren't too bad, but the sluice was different. The staff told me that it had to be perfect and that it would be inspected. Not only had the urine bottles and the bedpans to be sterilised using the correct solution, (unlike nowadays where the machines do the job,) but sometimes the items had to be scrubbed to the satisfaction of the nurse in charge. Then the commodes had to be dealt with, as also the sluice room itself, which had to be thoroughly washed down and absolutely immaculate for inspection!

Do you know what really galled me?

It was that you worked like mad, sweating buckets, expecting a visit from the charge nurse, (namely Frank in my case) and then after all of that work and worry he never turned up to inspect the work anyway. I thought that if I worked really hard Frank would come along and say, "Robert, you've done the most wonderful job, I've never seen the sluice looking so good. Congratulations!"

That never happened, I also reckon that the old timers kidded the students on to encourage them to do a good job, knowing that there wasn't going to be an inspection at all.

At the weekend there was more than the normal amount of visitors, there were a lot of concerned wives and other relatives, especially in the afternoon. I remember that one of the patients had a particularly lovely granddaughter. When Maurice realised this he became very interested and chatted to her, much to the consternation of Kat. Kat was very enamoured with Maurice and I think gave him a hard time over this, but he would shortly leave the ward anyway and he didn't take too much notice. He managed to arrange a date with this girl and they became heavily involved, whether or not it came to anything I don't know, but Kat found it hard to reconcile herself to their relationship and she was never quite the same afterwards.

I really felt sorry for some of the wives; because they told me so often that the husband that they had known and loved wasn't the same anymore. Not just because they were confused, but also often because the personality of the one they had loved and had lived with for so many years had changed. Sometimes a patient who presented to us as aggressive, had in earlier days been mild mannered and caring. There were some that swore and were short tempered, but the relatives told me that they had never sworn at all in their earlier lives.

There were many things that I learned as a student nurse on Devon ward. (Then, we weren't allowed to be addressed as nurse until we had completed our training and gained a qualification, till then we were always known as student nurse.) Not least among these things was the art of giving an enema. This again was something that wasn't on my own personal agenda, but it was in the curriculum and was necessary on a sick ward, because as much as the diet was on the whole adequate, the patients didn't get a great deal of exercise and often a lot of them had constipation.

I'm not sure whether it was a Saturday, or a Sunday job, but I am certain that it was something that we did at the weekend, and something that Henry seemed to rejoice in; rejoice in that is to say, because it was one of the procedures that needed to be taught to a student, and it was of course the most unwanted thing that was on the agenda, he seemed to enjoy my dislike of it.

I probably haven't mentioned the dreaded agenda for the student nurse. If we were to be successful as students, then we had to meet a certain criteria, this included getting a number of tasks ticked off in a little pink book, one of them being the care of the bowels. Every Saturday, or Sunday morning, Henry arranged, as was his normal custom to have a number of patients lined up on beds with curtains drawn around each one of course, and drawing a trolley alongside, with myself in attendance as his assistant, he commenced the dreadful deed.

There was a jug of water and soap on the trolley, along with a long rubber tube. In order to insert the tube in the appropriate place there had to be first a lubrication of the area then there had to be a rectal examination. Need I go on? The fact is that because the soapy water reached where the modern day phosphate enema doesn't always, there was almost without fail a good deal of success. Now this today may seem a little unnecessary, but it was in fact good nursing care then, if only for the reason that the confused patient, if he had an impacted bowel was liable to become even more confused and often aggressive too.

Anyway, moving on. One of the successes as a student that I was able to share in while staffed on Devon, was with a new patient, a tramp. This patient had been admitted during one of my weekends off. When I resumed for duty on the Monday morning Frank asked me to help him with this person, who, because of neglect was in an emaciated and disorientated state. We plied him with fluids and over a period of days encouraged him to eat.

The worst thing though was that he had scabies. Henry showed me the tracks that came up between his toes. In rather a concerned voice he said,

"We'll have to treat this, and then ourselves." Personally, I had never heard of scabies, so was unconcerned until Henry told me of the implications and exactly what it was. After that for several days, even though I had been treated I went around scratching myself while I worked, as did the rest of the staff, and writing now, as I recall it, I feel that I want to scratch again!

Fortunately the tramp recovered and after a couple of weeks was free to go on his way. But before he left Henry told me, "When you get a vagrant admitted as a patient you must search his clothes thoroughly, you see we often condemn them to be burned, but sometimes you will find hundreds of pounds hidden in them, particularly the lapels of his jacket."

It transpired that many tramps rolled the pound notes, or even the five and ten pound notes up, and then made a slit in the lapel, sliding the note down for safekeeping, then sewed the slit up again. Sometimes in the lining of the jacket there had been a small fortune found stashed away, though I think our own particular vagrant must have been a bit of a pauper.

He had been very nice nevertheless, and kind to the other patients when he started to feel better, and we rather missed him when he left; I remember very clearly waving him off as he made his way down the main road carrying a couple of plastic bags and a rucksack with him.

Despite myself and despite my misgivings, I had enjoyed myself on Devon ward, the work had been hard and frustrating, yet strangely enough, rewarding. I wondered though if I should really have been looking for a reward, perhaps I should have been satisfied that I was doing something for mankind that others may not have been able to do.

I have often heard the remark, 'I admire you, I couldn't do what you do.'

In fact I thought that I also wouldn't be able to do some of the things that I have been called upon to do, it just sort of turned out that way.

After a very quick three months on the ward, my time was coming to an end. I was sad, yet glad, and looked forward to my next placement with eager anticipation. Before that though I had to face Frank, who was obliged to fill in an assessment form for the nursing school, reflecting my performance over the past three months while on his ward. I needn't have been nervous because he gave me the best report that I had during my entire training.

"I'm probably going to get told off for this," Frank told me, "But as far as I'm concerned you deserve a good report, you've always tried to do your best and have never shirked, so I don't see how I can give you any less than this."

He pushed the completed report towards me to sign to say that I was happy with it.

I was never to receive such a report again, every place that could be 'ticked' as excellent was indeed, ticked. Not one of the others in my group got such a good report, either then, or later. I was really over the moon, I may not have been academic, but apparently I could nurse well, or at least I could nurse geriatrics well.

Finally before moving on, there is the matter of Henry's wig; did he ever wear it? The answer is yes, a couple of times. The theory among the staff was that he had made a new 'friend' and that he was seeing him after work, so he wanted to look his best. There were a few sniggers behind his back when he did choose to wear it, but not only didn't anyone want to hurt his feelings, but they were also afraid of the consequences if they were caught with a smirk on their faces, so we mostly ignored the wig. Henry looked markedly different on the occasions he wore it.

Chapter 8

If I were to put a title to this chapter I would call it 'The Matron.'

I felt that she the dreaded matron, merited a chapter all to herself. To myself and to many others who worked at St. Andrews and at hospitals throughout the country the matron was the only one of whom we were truly afraid. We were in awe of her, at least most of us were, the nursing officers were sometimes frightening, but the old type matron was different, even the other nursing officers held a great deal of respect for her. She was an institution, someone we had all read about, or seen in films as the fearsome ogre who ruled over the hospital like a tyrant.

I didn't know where to put this small chapter in the narrative, but although I wasn't able to place it earlier in the book, I didn't want to leave it too late.

There are what they call 'modern matrons' today and I'm sure they do a good job, but there was no one to compare with the old matron who instilled fear into the hearts of every nurse in the entire hospital, whichever hospital it might have been. She walked the wards until just before my training, when her title was changed to senior nursing officer. Nevertheless the change of name didn't change the awe and respect of the nursing staff towards her, despite her loss of status.

There were no matrons when I started nursing in 1974, there were only nursing officers and senior nursing officers, and the change had only recently been made. I personally thought that the nursing officers were threatening enough, but the old matron, who had been downgraded to one of the seniors, was terrifying.

A slim Irish woman with white hair made up into a bun, she was always immaculately dressed and wore the grey stockings that were essential to the uniform of the female nurse; almost as if she was making a statement, that even though she was stationed in the nursing office she was still very much a nurse and would ensure that high standards would be adhered to.

Miss O'Donnell was a spinster (I think that was almost obligatory for a matron) who had devoted her whole life to the nursing service. In her mid fifties, even her fellow nursing officers appeared to be in awe of her. She probably hadn't reconciled herself to the fact that she was no longer in sole control, at least of the female staff, (There was a matron for the female staff and a senior attendant responsible for the male staff in the old days) because, as I was told by one of the long serving nurses, matron was always in the fore when there was a problem to be solved.

There were stories of how the matron would come onto a ward and measure the distances between the beds and if they were an inch out she would severely reprimand the sister and the sister in turn would tear the junior staff to shreds. Sometimes the matron would surreptitiously wipe her fingers over the top of a curtain rail above any given bed and if there was dust on her fingers it went without saying that some junior nurse was in for the high jump.

These things didn't only happen on comedy films, they happened in real life and to the nursing staff they were very serious indeed. If matron came onto the ward any normal nurse would quake in her boots. Fortunately, though matron didn't do that sort of thing when I was training. Maybe because she was now only a mere nursing officer and felt that she had less power than previously, but maybe because anyway she had never been responsible for the male side in the past and she wasn't really interested.

I really don't know, all I know is that I was absolutely terrified of Miss O'Donnell. So of course were the rest of the staff; the female nurses in particular would be concerned that their caps were on straight and that the stiff collars with studs to keep them in place, which were part of the uniform in those days were always clean, or otherwise they knew that they were in serious trouble.

I remember one day I was sent to deliver a message to one of the nursing officers, but he wasn't there…. She was though!

"What is it you're wanting Mr. Panton?" She asked, in that brittle, threatening voice only a matron could use, and oh, so effectively! (Were they born that way?)

For the life of me I couldn't remember what it was I had come into the office for, and how did she know my name? I was absolutely non-plussed and terrified, and I really couldn't remember what I was there for, I don't recall how I got out of that situation, but I remember it to this day with embarrassment. Later I found out that she made it her business to know, not only the names of every single nurse in the hospital, but of every staff members whether catering, or cleaning staff, etc, etc, and there were hundreds of them.

She appeared formidable in appearance and so she was, but she also had a heart. One of the lads in my PTS. (Preliminary training school) was unfortunately stopped by the police and charged with drink driving. In those days that was a sackable offence, he expected instant dismissal, but because Miss O'Donnell learned that he had a wife and had been going through some difficulties in his marriage she intervened and he kept his job.

But apart from that, she was a devout Roman Catholic and whenever she came across a Catholic student, or indeed any member of the staff that was Roman Catholic by persuasion, she would round them up for Sunday mass and ensure, maybe under duress that they attended church on a Sunday, at the least.

Of course it goes without saying that if anyone had a problem and they needed any help her door was always open, but there were few that entered.

Personally I have to admit that I always had a sneaking admiration for her, although she scared me rigid. I felt that it must have been difficult for her to adjust to the new order of things, where nurses who were not overly qualified were promoted to nursing officers alongside her and although they weren't necessarily classed as the same grade, nevertheless they had almost the same standing.

Another incident that occurred regarding the matron happened one day while, as a second year student I was on an empty ward, the patients had all gone out to the rehab unit, or elsewhere and there was nothing to do. The charge nurse had disappeared to see one of his friends in another part of the hospital. I was at a loose end, so I sat down at a table and began to read the newspaper. It was delivered every day to each ward for the patients to presumably keep up with events in the outside world. I had only been there for a few seconds when, who should come through the door on her way to another ward, but the matron.

"Shouldn't you be doing something useful, like changing a bed, Mr. Panton?" she snapped as she hurried through.

"Yes, of course matron," I replied, guiltily.

Off I rushed to change a couple of beds. After that I thought the coast was clear so I sat down in the same place to recommence reading the newspaper. I could hardly believe my bad luck, when shortly after, matron again came back through, this time in the opposite direction and passed by me by without uttering a word!

The next day the nursing officer in charge of the ward visited and called me into the office. A nursing officer didn't usually invite students into the office, so I knew I was in trouble. To make it worse the person in question was Paddie O'Rourke with whom I had got on really well hitherto.

He was fuming.

"I've had a report that you're not doing your duties as well as you ought to be Mr. Panton, I'll have no slacking on my wards!"

And so he continued in the same vein for what seemed a very long time, making me well aware that he'd been given a dressing down and, that I in turn was receiving my just portion of it. Needless to say I was a very much more careful about any illicit activity that I undertook in the future!

I remember years later how I was for some reason running down a corridor in the hospital where I was then working. This was a cardinal sin, and as I turned a corner I bumped into the nursing officer.

He asked in a disapproving voice,

"Fire Mr. Panton, or Matron?"

Implicate in his enquiry was the fact that matron would most certainly not approve and he, who had been brought up under that regime didn't either.

When ‘matron’ retired a few years further into my career, I know that there were some that rejoiced and there were others who were relieved. There were some though, that like me felt sad, not just because Miss. O’Donnell was gone, but because it was an end of an era.

Chapter 9

During the next session in the classroom we were told that we were to have the opportunity to go and visit another hospital some miles up the road, where people with learning difficulties were looked after, actually it wasn’t called learning difficulties at the time, just then it was known as sub normality nursing, then later, mentally handicapped, the terms changed as society altered its attitude towards people who suffer with these ‘infirmities.’

It was nice to have a ride out to this hospital, which had once been a stately home. Smaller than St. Andrews, it was no less grand with magnificent grounds, but how upsetting it was to see these folk, that in many cases were in need of every basic thing that we take for granted, having to be supplied or catered for by the most dedicated of staff that I had ever come across up until that time. The thing that struck me most was the amount of patients who had Downs Syndrome, sadly in those days they were known as Mongols. These were the friendliest of all the patients there as I remember, and all of us students enjoyed talking with them and a number of us would play a game of snakes and ladders, or some other activity when requested.

Much later in my nursing career I thought that I would have a go at this type of nursing for a bit of a change; what a dreadful mistake I made!

The unit that I began my initiation in was a house that was the home to only five people, except that these people were children. Not so bad, one would think. Looking after four young boys and a girl, all of them about ten or eleven years old seemed quite appealing I imagined, before I took up the post; taking walks into town with them, or kicking a football around and generally enjoying myself while bringing some happiness to the children at the same time.

Sadly, it wasn't that simple, inasmuch as three of them were hyperactive, one was ok much of the time, but for no apparent reason he would begin throwing toys around the room and endangering anyone nearby with these missiles, the last of these youngsters was in a wheelchair and depended on the staff, (of which there were three on duty at any one time,) to do everything for him. The wheelchair had been adapted so that his legs, which he couldn't bend, could rest out before him without discomfort; it wasn't the sort of thing you could wheel around town without the possibility of causing someone an injury. Despite all of his problems including the inability to communicate, he seemed well aware of what was going on and everyone including myself was very fond of him.

Unfortunately the rest of the youngsters weren't as easy to deal with. One, the girl was very fond of the sister in charge of the unit and if she wasn't there for any reason this girl would shout and bawl and cause general mayhem around the house, requiring at least two of the three nurses to be in attendance on her when this behaviour occurred. Of course she didn't behave like this all the time, it only seemed like all the time, to me at least. We used every tactic that we could think of to distract her when she was behaving in this way, but usually with little result.

There was one thing that I noticed though; those nurses had the patience of a saint. Nothing seemed to annoy, or fluster them, and nothing was too much trouble, they loved those children, whereas I found myself getting rattled inside and didn't know what to do next to keep them happy. Their attention span was so short I found myself always thinking of the next move in an attempt to keep the house quiet and peaceful, and the challenging children contented.

There was one of the youngsters who ran around the house whilst shouting at the top of his voice, for no apparent reason other than to release his energy, and quite often he was put out into the enclosed garden to help him to burn his excess energy off, as he careered around and around shouting with all his might, goodness knows what the neighbours must have thought about it, but we never seemed to get any complaints from them.

One of the children, the toy thrower, was usually quite content if someone would sit with him and read a book, he would find it really fascinating to look at the pictures and for one of the staff to explain any simple story to him.

The last one I remember is the one who was the reason for my begging the general manager to find me a new post. He was a nice lad, although he had learning difficulties he was quite easy to manage most of the time, except for the day that I was asked by the sister to give him an enema. I thought that it would be simple,

'No problem, I've done it dozens of times,' I thought.

So off I went to fetch a micro enema and calling this young man upstairs to his bedroom, I commenced to take down his trousers. I should have seen the warning signs of disapproval, but I didn't. As I began to insert what was a very small tube into his rectum all hell broke loose! He began by trying to bite me; as a result I started to hold him around his waist; big mistake! He then began to tear at my shirt, a new one by the way, and then, after that seeing that I was still clinging on, he began to scratch me on my chest. I'm not talking about little scratches here, but about the type of scratches that a Siamese cat gives to those who take it to the vets unwillingly.

Well what was I to do? I let go, of course and sheepishly made my way down the stairs to report my failure to the sister, who though sympathetic, couldn't help but giggle, as did the other nurse on duty; I don't blame them, what a sight I must have looked!

As it was nearly time for me to end my shift I asked the most understanding sister to let me go home to nurse my wounds.

I had had enough; one month, or thereabouts, of torture during that time, where I went home to my wife in a bad mood after every shift, and dreaded each day that dawned, knowing that I had to face it all again; I just couldn't do it any more.

I begged my general manager,

"Please, put me somewhere else! I can't stand it anymore. If you don't, I'll have to leave the unit and the hospital trust."

After hearing my tale of woe, he did without argument move me, albeit to a hospital which catered for the elderly mentally ill, something that I didn't really want to do, but it was ten thousand times better than working with those children. It isn't that I didn't like the children; each one was a little individual who needed love and understanding, and an awful lot of patience. I just wasn't cut out for it; each person has their skills and their limitations and I knew that I wasn't able to cope. There is one thing though in all of this. I saw how those nurses dealt with their very difficult patients, and their dedication was beyond anything that I had seen before, ever! They loved their charges and would cuddle and cosset them, even though they often got nothing in return. If anyone in the health service deserved a gold medal, they did, each and every one looking after such needy people; in fact I could almost call those staff saintly, they were beautiful people!

All of that was a long way into the future, meanwhile on the way home from the mental handicapped hospital in the coach we all agreed that it had been an experience that we would never forget and as we turned into the drive of St. Andrews we went our ways home, or to the social club having had our eyes opened to a world that few of us had realised existed.

The fortnight in school passed quickly, as we learned about the different types of schizophrenia and some of the various medicines that were used to alleviate the symptoms. We went further into things like the difference between psychosis and neurosis, acute and chronic states.

It was the neurotic illnesses that I was particularly interested in, anxiety and its causes and the different types of depression and the reason why some people suffered from it.

There was the inevitable end of block test of course, which I again passed with a miserably low mark. After the test we all hurried to the notice board to find out where our next placement would be. Mine was at Salisbury House, a large building standing apart from the main hospital, though still within the grounds.

It had originally been built in the thirties as a TB. ward and at the back it had a huge conservatory attached to it. Not knowing what to expect when I started on Monday morning I asked Raj what he thought as he had been assigned there on his first placement.

"You will either like it, or hate it," he said,

"The charge nurse doesn't much like first year students, because they haven't got a lot of experience and he thinks that they get in the way.

I didn't like him and I don't think that he liked me much either." He said in a sombre sort of way.

Well that really cheered my weekend up no end. Not only that thing about the charge nurse, but I also found out that it was a ward of about fifty patients and all middle aged, or elderly schizophrenics.

Would I ever get to work among the younger element, those who would sit on a bench with me and pour out their troubles, so that I could be of some real use?

Chapter 10

As I parked my car on the Monday morning I could see the lights on in the downstairs windows of Salisbury house. It was a large building, as it had to hold fifty patients. To me, in the darkness of the winter's morning it had an air of foreboding. I was nervous as usual and it took some effort to prise myself out of my nice warm car and make the hundred yard walk to the ward.

Walking slowly up the short drive to the front door, I could see through the Georgian type windows. It was a high ceilinged, gloomy looking place with the walls painted in gloss paint that looked rather as if it had been done twenty years or more ago. I put my key into the door, only to find that it wouldn't turn in the lock. Apparently there were male and female keys, not that all of the female keys fitted female wards and vice versa, because over the years the wards had changed their occupancy many times. Still I had the wrong type of key, so I rang the doorbell. No reply! I tried again; still no joy. It transpired that the doorbell didn't work.

I began to knock on the door, but I knew that I probably wouldn't have any success as the main door opened onto a staircase, with another door a little way down a corridor, and that was closed, so no one could hear me.

Fortunately a patient came down the stairs as I stood knocking futilely and he went to fetch someone to let me in. After a couple of minutes a male nurse (They all seemed to be men on that ward,) came sauntering up to the door and let me in. This same nurse it transpired was leaving that day to commence a career in the outside world. When he learned about my situation re. the key he gave me his own. I was now in the unusual and enviable position of having in my possession both a male and a female key. I'll never know how that nurse got away without having to pay for the key that he gave me.

I needn't have worried about the charge nurse that morning, as it was his day off, instead the staff nurse Ron was in charge of the shift. I had never met anyone quite like him; he was full of life and joviality. Aged about thirty, I later found that he was married to a lovely lady.

I couldn't understand how he had captured such a beauty, as he was very ugly and scruffy even in his hospital suit. He wore gold rimmed spectacles with extremely thick lenses that usually looked as if they needed a good clean, yet there he was married to a lovely looking woman. I assumed that it was his personality that did it!

Ron had the filthiest sense of humour that I'd ever come across. Nevertheless I liked him instantly. He was warm and kind as he introduced me to the rest of the staff.

"Right lads," he said after the night staff had gone home. "Let battle commence!"

Upstairs the half dozen of us proceeded to get the majority of the patients up for their breakfast. Some were already downstairs, but the ones that were left needed some 'assistance.' When I say assistance I don't mean the sort of help that we gave the patients on Devon ward. This was quite different.

Because we were away from the main building and therefore out of the sight of authority, I'm afraid that anything went in Salisbury House.

The mode of getting the patients out of bed was variable; some would co operate and that was alright, they were the lucky ones. Others were rather resistive and wanted to lie in. This wasn't allowed, so those who could be dragged out of bed and dressed were quite literally dragged out of their beds.

Others were made of sterner stuff, or so they thought. These were tipped slowly off their mattresses, just enough to allow them time to scramble out before they hit the floor so they wouldn't hurt themselves, then they were unwillingly dressed while still wiping the sleep from their eyes.

There was one who was quite different from the rest, this was Kenny and the modus operandi for him was to take his shoes, which were parked under his bed and then run like fury. It never failed, if he wouldn't get out of his bed the answer was to simply take his shoes. He could run alright, and run he did, to try and catch the culprit. I tried it once later on and nearly came a cropper. He didn't take any prisoners if you had his shoes in your possession, he would certainly beat you to a pulp if he caught you. The secret was to race around the ward, down one staircase, along the bottom corridor, through the dayroom and then along the other corridor, up the stairs and then replace the shoes underneath his bed again. By the time he had chased the nurse bold enough to take on this task he was so exhausted that he was like a lamb and could be dressed without fear of retaliation. He was just satisfied that he had his shoes back in his possession. I know that this tale sounds incredible, but it's absolutely true and the beauty of it was that no one would tell you off for running!

Why were the staff so eager to get everyone up in such a hurry?

Well one of the reasons was that there were so many patients and so few staff; I think that there were six on duty at any one time and I don't believe that was adequate to meet all of the patients needs. Nevertheless that's how it was and maybe it's the case now, wards always running below the staffing levels needed to do the job properly.

Unfortunately in this case there was another reason for the rush, which quite disgustingly was that the staff wanted to get breakfast over and done with so they could have their own. They didn't care so much about the patients, but more about themselves.

In Salisbury House there were a lot of hungry patients, but there were also a few hungry staff as well and the patients were given the minimum amount of eggs and bacon, etc, so that there was enough left over for the staff to have their illicit share, indeed the staff had their meals plated up first sometimes, and then put into the hot plate to be eaten after the inconvenience of seeing to the patients beforehand. They didn't get the small amount that the patients received. I think that their plates represented the lions share!

It is true that over the years I also ate the patients food, which if you were caught meant instant dismissal, so went the story, but I never knew anyone who was sacked for it and the practice was rife throughout the hospital. I did make it a rule to only eat what was left over after all the patients had dined and were fully satisfied. In fact if there were any leftovers they would either go to the pigs, or down the waste disposal unit, so I never felt too guilty about taking the food the patients didn't want.

What was going on here though was different; the staff were taking food from hungry patients and eating it themselves. In fairness this was the only ward that I saw this practice going on and although there were also other things I saw that I was unhappy with, I never blew the whistle, I was a first year student, raw and unsure of myself. I truly believed that if I said anything the others would close ranks and deny it, or that I would be ostracised, so sadly I took the cowards way out and said nothing, to my everlasting shame.

Funnily enough on Salisbury before the meals were served a large bell was rung, it swung to and fro, just like the one that the metalwork teacher had used when I was at school, as we were called in from our playtime. It seemed to herald a veritable feast, but here in fact it rang to bring the patients, at least sometimes to a virtual famine.

When the staff's breakfast, which was taken at a leisurely pace, was over, it was time for shaving the patients. Some of them were able to do this for themselves, but the vast majority of them had to be seen to by the staff. Not Ron of course, he was the staff nurse and did nothing much if he could help it. The task had to be undertaken by myself as a first year student, and two or three others, usually nursing assistants, or second year students, sometimes a combination of the two.

I doubt that many who read this have attempted to shave something like thirty men in a matter of an hour, but it was not a job for the faint hearted. For one thing I wasn't exactly adept at the art, although I had shaved quite a number on Devon ward, but the shaving equipment wasn't quite like we have today.

What a mess some of them looked afterwards, with cuts all over their faces a lot of the time. You see they weren't like the average man that would pop into the barbers shop and sit perfectly still in the knowledge that the man doing the job was competent, not a bit of it. Many of the patients sat down, or some stood in fear and trepidation of what was to come, especially if a newcomer like myself was on the scene. They would sometimes have a nervous tick, or be restless due to their illness, or medication and it was, to say the very least a difficult job.

One of the patients in particular was to be avoided at all costs if it were possible, that was Reggie who always seemed to have a runny nose, I don't want to go into details, suffice it to say that it was always a mucky job with him.

We constantly had to change the blades and one after another patient appeared at the door in a seemingly never-ending stream. It was always a job that if we could get out of, then we would. Rather do the bed making was the call of the day, and that was a massive job in itself. Still, once the shaving was over the morning seemed quite relaxed in comparison to the frenzy of the first couple of hours.

The next thing that occurred was giving out the cigarettes. This was a sight to see, there were perhaps thirty of the patients who smoked. One of them was Reggie, the one with the runny nose. He was a small ugly and dirty looking man of about seventy. If he could steal a cigarette, or even a butt end off another patient he would, without qualm or hesitation.

"Hey, kid. Hey kid, give us a bit. Hey, kid. Hey kid, give us a bit." He'd call out constantly, spitting on the ground meanwhile and looking with eagle eyes for a sign of any patient who would be careless enough either to drop their cigarette, or be stupid enough to stub it out half way through and put the tab end behind his ear; an easy target for Reggie!

Then there was Terry a man of about sixty years of age who years before had had a leucotomy, which was an operation that was done on the brain to relieve tension in someone who was tormented by his illness, such as a person who was becoming hostile, or violent, because of perhaps, obsessional behaviour, or because he was hearing voices that caused him great distress, and sometimes I believe due to severe depression. A hole or maybe two were drilled into the top of his forehead as part of the procedure, and Terry had the tell tale signs of two small dents in his forehead. Perhaps at one time they would have been hidden by his hair, but now he was balding and they were very evident. Terry was very placid, even docile, but he did like his cigarettes and the only time that I saw him animated was when they were given out. He would protect his cigarette as if it were the crown jewels. Reggie didn’t stand a chance with him.

Another patient that I came to love was Ernie, he would wander around, or sit looking very morose. I sat with him sometimes to see if I could get some conversation from him, but all he would keep on saying was,

"Sadness, its all sadness you see," without telling me what exactly he felt sad about.

That was the frustrating thing, I had been in nursing for several months now, but I had never been able to have a single worthwhile conversation with a patient to find out what made them tick and what made them feel the way they did, or how they arrived at that state the they were in.

While I was watching this ritual of the cigarette distribution for the first time, Ron who was in charge of the proceedings, (after all it was a job that didn't need a lot of effort,) asked Carl, who was a third year student to show me around the ward on that first day.

Carl was a man of about the same age as myself and despite the fact that he worked very hard all the time that I was on the ward, doing the shaving and bathing, and all the other things that were required of us lesser mortals, (students I mean,) he always seemed to look immaculate, he was about six feet tall, wore glasses and sported a different tie every day.

Salisbury and Devon were as different as chalk is from cheese. The whole place seemed shabby, and was set out on two floors. The walls of the lower floor wore a yellow tinge from all the

cigarette smoke. The ward had two staircases, one each side of the building, the kitchen being in the corridor on one side and the office and the bathroom where all the shaving was done were on the other.
Next to the office corridor there were partitions dividing all the various rooms and corridors up, these had glazed panels in each of them, so you could stand at one end of the ward, yet still see right through to the other. There was a large day room divided into two in the same manner, and then the huge conservatory, which I mentioned before. All the floors throughout the building were wooden, as opposed to the tiled floors of Devon ward.

Certainly there was enough room for all the patients to have their own space, and indeed there seemed to be some that always chose to sit in one area and others that would mill around in another. Those who wanted to get away from the others often went into the dining room, situated next to the kitchen. They could be assured of a bit of peace and quiet here, as most of the others hung around at the other end of the ward, waiting like vultures to pounce when one of the frequent cigarette rounds occurred.

In the room nearest the office there was a television that I was to find out later was rarely turned on except in the evenings and at weekends sometimes, it was mostly watched by the staff, especially if there was a football match on at the weekend, or a particularly good film thought to be worth watching. Also, there was a table tennis table, which was to be my salvation, whilst on this placement, although I didn't know it then.

There seemed to be very few other activities that the patients could take part in except for a few board games. When later I attempted to lure a few of them into playing some of those games though, no one was interested. I did manage to get one of them to play chess with me once, but it was only once, after that he refused. Was I really that bad?

To be fair there were occupational therapists and voluntary workers who came in from time to time and threw a ball around to a disinterested few, or would try and tempt the patients with some sort of activity, but I'm afraid with most of them it was like flogging a dead horse, unless a cigarette was on offer they didn't really want to know.

As we made our way upstairs I talked to Carl about the patients.

"Are all of them schizophrenics?" I asked.

"Most of them," he told me, "They're what is unofficially termed, 'burnt out schiz's,' though don't mention that in the school, or they'll throw you out! The acute symptoms that you'll see in a young person who's been recently diagnosed, often subside as the years go by, and they end up like these people. All they care about is where the next fag's coming from and when is the next meal; they like their grub."

I hesitated before I asked the next question; yet felt that I had to ask it anyway.

"If," I asked hesitantly, "They like their food, then why do the staff eat some of it? I didn't think there was really enough to go around anyway, this morning."

Carl looked around before answering.

"Look," he said, with a soft voice, "This ward's separated from the others and because it's quite isolated it has its own rules. Tony, (that was the name of the charge nurse,) does his own thing, he leaves Ron to run the show. Quite a lot of the time he isn't around, he's either visiting his mates, or having a kiss and a cuddle in the office with one of the domestics, who you'll see sneaking onto the ward every so often. I know that the food thing isn't right and at first I wouldn't join in, but I realised it wouldn't make any difference if I didn't. Anything that the staff leave is thrown into the pig bin, even if the patients are on short rations. If you rock the boat you'll regret it; the nursing officer is one of Tony's mates and sometimes sneaks over here himself to get something to eat."

I felt miserable, what had I come to?

Afterwards I realised that though some of the nurses in charge were a law unto themselves the great majority were only concerned with the welfare of their patients, Tony just wasn't one of them. He was a bad leader and the other staff just followed his lead. There were several patients who later told me that they were afraid of him and were always glad when it was his day off. What an indictment on his professionalism.

Anyway, we toured the upstairs, where there were several dormitories, each partitioned off in the same way as down below, so that more or less anywhere that a nurse stood he could see what was going on throughout the entire floor. I noticed that the state of the wards cleanliness left something to be desired. I imagine that was something to do with the fact that if the charge nurse wasn't bothered, neither would the domestic staff be. They had two of these domestics on duty during the daytime.

Upstairs, as downstairs there was a bathroom and toilet area, but the only bathroom that was active during the day was the one downstairs, where every afternoon seven, or so of the patients were given a bath, each getting one a week.

As we went down to the day room again there was a patient sitting on the steps, Carl introduced me to Walter, who apparently sat there most of the time. He didn't smoke and liked his own company, so chose to spend most of his day there.

"Do you like it here?" he asked me.

I told him that I was a little nervous because it was so new to me.

"Oh, you don't want to worry," he said loudly, "What's the use of worrying? There's no need to worry," he continued, his voice rising higher in volume and in pitch as he finished each phrase,

"Its no good worrying, we're all going to die one day, but if you've got to go, you've got to go, there's no good worrying about it!"

Carl beckoned me away, and after we were out of earshot he told me that Walter always spoke in the same manner, and Ron loved to get him to a point of frenzy, where he would begin to slap at the wall, because he'd become overexcited.

Back in the dayroom the patients were wandering around aimlessly, some with a fixed stare, others sometimes chatting in a fashion, or annoying one another, others sat with vacant faces, in the chairs that lined the walls.

There were two things that I noticed at that time, one was the shocking state of their clothes, they were either too small, or too large, often the trouser legs were too short, and invariably the smoking brigade had burn holes all over their trousers and jackets, yes I believe that most of them wore jackets, which seemed strange to me, they weren't going anywhere after all were they, as all the doors were kept permanently locked! Personally I thought that it would have been more appropriate to have them wearing cardigans, or jumpers, and no jackets, but I daren't say so.

The other thing I noticed was the aggression and hostility among some of them, their language was colourful to say the least, and a few of them, were much worse than the others, it didn't bother me though, because in my youth I was famous for my foul mouth.

Later on in my placement there, one of the patients had a disagreement with another, probably over a cigarette, there were a few choice words spoken, then the first patient hit the second with such force that he died a little later, I wasn't on duty that day, but there were many times that I and the rest of the staff had to break up a fight. The patient who was the perpetrator of this act seemed to have a had little group all of his own and I felt afraid of him, although I was told by Ron not to show fear in front of any of the patients, as they would take this as a sign of weakness and play on it. That was perhaps the best advice that he ever gave me and it stood me in good stead over the years.

Funnily enough with all this underlying aggression going on I don't remember any patient threatening a member of staff, perhaps Ron had given them all the same advice. Not of course that all the patients were like this, many of them were quiet and retiring, much of the trouble that did come along was to do with cigarettes that were handed out so regularly. If the staff didn't want to feed the patients properly, at least they managed to cater for them in this area, mind you it did make the place smell; it certainly wasn't a healthy environment!

The rest of that shift was spent in observing the patients and then serving lunch. There were quite a few Polish men and one Russian on the ward, apparently they had been prisoners of war and had become mentally ill, I imagine because of the trauma's of war. These were amongst the quietest of the patients, often keeping to their own little groups and doing most things for themselves. Some of them helped to lay the tables at mealtimes and cleared away the dirty dishes afterwards.

The medicine round was a mammoth task and I was asked to help with this, with Carl telling me something about each tablet and liquids that he dished out and as I took them to the various individuals.

After the lunch was over it was time for handover, which again, as on Devon ward only the senior nurses attended.

The patients got their full quota of food at lunch time because we were all due to go off duty afterwards, so the staff didn't have a need to take any of it, except maybe the odd mouthful!

There was one bright note on this, my first and rather depressing day.

Bert who had been in the hospital a staggering fifty years was discharged. I don't know where he went, all I know is that he left with mixed feelings. He had a smile on his face, but I'm sure that he must have been sad and concerned inside. After all he had been there longer than all the staff in the hospital, and probably longer than any other patient. I wish now that I had taken more notice of where he was going to, even more than that, I would liked to have read his notes to find out why he was admitted in the first place. There didn't seem to be anything wrong with him. He spoke absolutely rationally and seemed quite 'normal.' A man in his seventies, I would guess. The only thing I noticed that was different about him, as far as I could see, was that he had what was called then, a club foot, and as a result he wore one of those built up boots attached to a calliper. I just hope that he was happy wherever he went.

Chapter 11.

The next day I arrived at the required time and let myself into the ward. Most of the other staff were already there and were having a cup of tea before beginning the daily routine. The charge nurse, Tony was in the office taking the handover and I didn't meet him until later that morning, after the shaving had been done.

I had been standing around observing the patients, when one of them came up to me and asked if I would play table tennis with him. I had never played the game in my life and as it happened neither had the patient, judging by the mess we made of things.

"Shouldn't you be doing something productive?" a voice called out from the direction of the office.

I stood stock still not knowing who was speaking and who he was speaking to. Turning around after a moment, I discovered that it was Tony and the object of his question was myself. He was a well built athletic man a few years older than me, he looked stern then and even afterwards, when I got to know him better I thought he looked a bit threatening and he was always rather serious even when he was with the staff he got on well with.

"I'm sorry," I muttered, feeling rather anxious after what I had heard about him.

"The patient wanted to play table tennis."

"Well, if that's the best you can do, you would be better off making some beds, or sorting the linen cupboard out," he said sarcastically.

"Come on then," he continued, having thought for a moment,

"Let's see if we can do something with you. By the way, what's your name, you're my new student, aren't you?"

I told him that I was and gave him my name and also said that I didn't know a thing about table tennis, but he wasn't listening, he served a ball in my direction, which of course I missed. Then, he began to show me how to serve.

"The art of table tennis is knowing how to serve well," he explained.

For the next hour instead of making beds, or observing the patients with their cigarettes, I played table tennis. 'What a way to earn a living,' I said to myself later, on the way home.

Every day that I went into work, after the main tasks of the shift were done, there was Tony waiting to teach me more about the game, until I actually became quite a good player. I was careful of course not to win too many of our matches, because I knew on which side my bread was buttered!

Some of the other staff became quite annoyed because I wasn't doing the work that I should have been, and of course they weren't able to skive off with him as they usually did; one or two of them being part of his little club. But, there was really very little I could do about it, Tony wanted me to play and how could I say no?

This went on throughout my placement, except for the times when he entertained his young lady in the office, or went off to see one of his friends on another ward. I confess that I was quite put out by his breaks away, especially as, having got to know him so well now, I was able to say things to him that most of the other staff couldn't. I teased him when he dropped a shot and took the mickey out of him occasionally; he seemed to lap it up. At times, I was even invited into his office and sat talking to him for hours at a time, until one day the nursing officer came in unexpectedly and found me in there and Tony was asked to inform me that it wasn't acceptable. Even though the nursing officer was his friend, protocol had to be abided by, he wouldn't confront me himself of course, one of the ways that the nursing officers retained their awesome reputation was by getting others to tell the students off, and thereby seeming more threatening.

I have to admit that I felt embarrassed by all the attention that I was getting from Tony, and on top of that I wasn't doing my job properly, or learning from my experience on the ward, yet I felt powerless to resist, to me it was a matter of survival. I didn't like the man, but I knew that if I upset him things could become very difficult for me. Nevertheless, he wasn't always on duty and often when he was he had to concern himself with other things. Those were the times that I worked alongside the others, or sat with the patients and got to know them.

One of the favourites on the ward was Kenny he was a man in his late sixties and was the one who would chase his shoes in the morning, if it became necessary to use that method to get him out of bed. If anyone asked him how he was he would reply,

"I'm not so well, I got my hand caught in mothers mangle," and he would show you his left hand, the tips of his fingers being indeed rather flat.

It appears that when he was a lad he took a fancy to putting his hand into the mangle his mother was using to squeeze the water out of some clothing. A mangle by the way, for the uninitiated, was a hand turned pair of rollers that was used by the housewives of Kenny's day to get the excess water out of the washing before hanging it on the line.

Kenny was a very laid back sort of person unless he felt that there was something that merited some exertion, such as chasing his shoes. Apart from the thing about the mangle he really had very little to say. I remember only two things, one was that if he was out for a walk, and we occasionally took him out for a breath of air; whatever the weather he would always say,

"Cold, in'it?"

The perspiration might be pouring down his face, but it was always "Cold in'it?"

There was something more delicate and potentially embarrassing Kenny would say and do, if he got the opportunity. The ladies who would visit the ward, mostly at the weekend were the wives, or daughters of the patients and they were only too aware of the type of patients that we had on Salisbury, some of them had been visiting for years, so if Kenny approached them they knew what to expect.

"Let me feel your dugs Mrs." he would say, while reaching out to touch one of their breasts.

"Get away with you Kenny, you dirty old man." Would be a typical response, while the female in question invariably wore an affectionate smile on her face.

Unfortunately staff nurse Ron, whose sense of humour was of the less savoury type, took things too far one day. There was an invitation for some of the staff and patients to attend some sort of conference in the hospital. For Ron it was too much of an opportunity to be missed, so he asked me to accompany him, along with Kenny and another quite inoffensive patient.

We arrived before the venue was full and Ron sat Kenny next to a stern, prim and proper looking social worker. The proceedings began after a few minutes, but as Ron predicted within a short space of time Kenny, being no doubt bored turned to this lady and said in a rather loud voice,

"Can I feel your dugs, Mrs?" he asked, groping for her breasts as he spoke.

The lady let out an almighty scream and jumped from her chair, her face red and flustered and not knowing where to put herself.

Well, I nearly lost control of myself, how I stopped myself from bursting out laughing I don't know, certainly I was shaking and was in an agony in an attempt to prevent a squeal of hysterics from bursting through my firmly closed lips.

Ron was in deep trouble and even though our nursing officer, when he heard about it thought it was as hilarious as everyone else, he had to go through the motions of giving Ron a good dressing down. I really believe that that particular prank slowed down Ron's promotion to charge nurse by several years; in fact I became a charge nurse myself, long before he ever did.

I'd like to tell you one more little story Just before I leave the subject of Kenny, who by the way was held in great affection by all the staff, even Tony.

One day I was asked to take him out somewhere, I don't remember where and it doesn't matter, but we had to be there at a particular time. No one had told me though that Kenny had an obsession, he had to kick every lamp post and every tree along the route. After a few of these 'kicking's' I was getting a bit fed up, knowing that we were running late. In an effort to speed thing up I told him in no uncertain terms that he had to stop kicking everything in sight. He persisted of course, and I, getting a little irate by this time attempted to pull him away from the next tree, Kenny took a swing at me and became angry, so I naturally let him have his own way. We were late for our appointment of course, and worse still I had to endure it all again on the way back to the ward.

I know that in this chapter and in the preceding one I have said some rather cutting things about the staff and the practices on Salisbury, but I want to make it clear before I go any further that the nursing staff on there weren't all bad; of course most of them were really caring people. Even Ron, who liked a laugh and sometimes baited the patients because he liked to see the reaction, actually was very kind to the patients most of the time. Tony though, would treat them as if they were boys in a borstal, shouting at them from one end of the ward to the other, if he thought that something untoward was going on. Not that occasionally they didn't need firm handling, of course they did, by the very nature of their mental state and the fact that so many of them were confined in one relatively small space. At times, as a result there was a lot of tension on the ward.

A few of them were allowed out on their own for a walk and others went out daily to the 'so called' rehabilitation centre, where we as students spent a couple of mind numbing weeks during our training, helping the patients to snap together plastic containers, or put bottles of perfume into boxes.

Rehabilitation?

It was enough to drive anyone crazy, and we all hated it. Still, I suppose it served a purpose for the patients who received a very small wage at the end of the week.

There was one patient that I was very fond of while I was there, Roland, an older man who was always very placid and although he wandered around the ward mingling with the others he was in fact a loner, he didn't smoke and therefore didn't get into the middle of any of the rumpuses that sometimes went on over cigarettes. After a few weeks though, his behaviour changed, he became very vocal and would go up to one, or another of the patients and use foul language at them for no reason, some took exception to this and as a result he received one or two punches. Whether this is what caused him to become physically ill I don't know, but he stopped eating and after a while became thin and emaciated and was so weak that he just sat in a chair staring into space, not saying a word. When this had gone on for some time he was transferred to Devon ward, where he eventually died.

Another patient likewise began to show extreme aggression, but this time he used physical violence against some of the others. He was young and well built and although the doctor prescribed him extra medication, to such a point that his speech was slurred, he continued to be aggressive towards both patients and eventually the staff. This man was secluded in a side room upstairs and a member of staff was on duty outside of the locked door at all times, while he kicked and shouted from within the room.

Eventually it was decided that he would have to go to a secure hospital, but this took weeks to arrange, and he was still in seclusion when I finished my time on the ward. It was quite a scary thing taking him his meals and emptying his commode. Two or three nurses had to be with him when anything like this had to be done. We often had to restrain him, as at that point in time restraining techniques weren't taught to the staff, it was a bit hit and miss, to say the least. I'm not particularly well built, so I was always nervous at these times, both with this patient and with others that I met like him afterwards.

There was another incident with a patient who was to be discharged out into the community while I was on the ward, he didn't want to leave; he had been in Salisbury for several months, one of only a handful of patients who hadn't been there for many years. When it came to getting him ready for discharge he refused to get dressed

"I'm not leaving, I like it here," he protested.

Albert was usually a very placid man, but he began to get resistive when a nursing assistant and I tried to persuade him to co-operate.

"Come on," I said," it's no good stalling, you've been told by the doctor that you've got to leave, after all its got to be better than staying here."

“You don’t understand,” he said, “I’ve made some really good mates here and I want to stay, cant you do something to help me?”

I went to call for help, and Ron and Carl came upstairs to the dormitory. Ron, who usually had quite a good relationship with Albert, sat on the bed and explained why he had to get ready to leave. At first Albert responded, but halfway through being dressed, having only his shirt on and nothing down below, he got up from the bed and made a dash for it. Ron and Carl caught him before he could get too far, but Albert continued to struggle and in the process caught his backside on one of the old fashioned radiators that were situated under some of the windows all around the ward. The radiator was hot, very hot, and Albert let out a loud yell as the heat burned the top layer of skin off his buttocks. We all felt really sorry about this, but as he was compliant now, the process of dressing was finished off.

When he was downstairs Ron took him into the clinic and treated the burn, and so Albert was discharged a little later. How sad that he had to go under such circumstances. Whether or not Ron had to face the music for this incident, I don’t remember, but in all fairness, it wasn’t done on purpose. Unfortunately the whole event wasn’t handled well and Albert suffered as a result.

As I mentioned earlier the doors on Salisbury and the vast majority of the other wards were locked. There were probably about thirty wards and villas in all, and each had their own reason for restricting their patients. On Salisbury most of them were kept in for their own safety, but volunteer visitors took some of them out frequently, or if there were enough staff they were taken out by the students, or nursing assistants.

Much later, I worked in another hospital looking after the elderly mentally ill. While I was there they brought in a system whereby if you wanted to enter or leave the ward you pressed a button that would deactivate the door alarms. The door was kept unlocked, so as to theoretically, at least give the impression that the patients weren't prisoners. If one of them walked out without pressing the button, the alarm would sound and the patient would be coaxed back in. If he were a 'sectioned' patient there was no problem, but if he wasn't and he resisted verbal persuasion, then the nurses would take him by the arm and bring him back. Technically if the patient resisted and had to be forced back in, then I think this may have, in the eyes of the law been classed as assault.

In my opinion, having a system like that is the same as having a locked door. Indeed some of the nurses in charge locked it anyway, because the unlocked door tied up staff that were obliged to go chasing out after any persistent offenders who constantly tried to abscond. The reason why the door needed to be locked was that not far away was a main road and the patient, sometimes in a pair of pyjamas would wander up the street and was in danger of either catching his death of cold, or being knocked down by a car. We weren't trying to imprison the patients, but due to their confusion, we were attempting to give them a safe environment. I will never understand why the powers that be couldn't see that argument!

Anyway, now I've come down from my hobbyhorse, I'll continue!

In the last few days of my time there, Tony wanted to close the ward down, because there was a cricket match in the hospital grounds and he wanted to watch it. He thought that it would be a good idea if everyone went, so he despatched them all in groups with a nurse in charge of each little band of unwilling would be spectators. Not many of them really wanted to go, but Tony was determined.

One of the last to protest was a tall, hefty man who was usually quiet and never a problem, but this time he took a stand against Tony's rule of law. He was adamant that he wasn't going to go.

"I don't even like the game," he protested.

Tony was really angry!

"You're going to do as you're told, whether you like it or not!" came the furious reply.

There were harsh words flying about on both sides, Tony, in a rage caught the offender by his tie and read him the riot act. In the ensuing struggle the patient fell backwards with Tony sprawling on top of him. Whilst on the floor he began to show the patient more aggression than he should have, (of course, he shouldn't have shown him any at all.) and one of the other nurses standing there waiting to leave the ward, pulled him off.

"You're going too far, Tony, get up before you get yourself into trouble," he warned.

Tony realised that he had overstepped the mark and panting got up, and then helped the patient to his feet. Strangely enough the patient decided that he would go after all and Tony got his wish, the ward was locked and left empty as we went away to the cricket match.

Not long after I had left Salisbury ward Tony got a job as a nursing officer in another part of the country. The next time that I worked there a new and much pleasanter man had been put in charge. It seemed strange to me that Tony could be promoted, when most of the people in the hospital knew what he was like, but there again, perhaps that's why he moved away, knowing that he was likely to be overlooked for promotion at St.

Andrews. I didn't understand what had happened with him, surely he must have started out with good intentions, but somewhere along the line he lost his way.

Chapter 12

Before our next placement the P.T.S. group were given a fortnights holiday. We weren't allowed to choose the timing of the holiday, much to the anger of some of the group, but that was what it was like in those days, you just did as you were told!

We ambled along to the old notice board first of all, to see where we were going to be placed next. I was quite excited when I realised that I was going to an admission ward until someone informed me that it wasn't an 'acute' admission ward, but a ward that catered for re admissions. In other words those patients that had been in hospital previously and had been discharged, but had broken down again, and in some cases again and again. It wasn't quite the same as Salisbury, but with some of the same patients it was verging on it, though I was to find that there would be the odd first time admission, so actually it didn't turn out as bad as I thought it would be as I went away for a break.

It was a nice holiday, and besides the weather at that time of the year (the month of May,) we all enjoyed it, my wife, two children and myself. We went over to France, where, I remember an old lady in Calais told me off for dropping some litter, much to my shame. When we returned to Dover, after only one day, (well that was all I could afford on my meagre salary!) there was a mist like one of those old pea souper's that we had when I was a boy and we pitched the tent in the dark murkiness; happily we were to wake up in the morning to a glorious day.

Ah, well, the holiday was all over now and I found myself standing outside Stafford ward one sunny afternoon, wishing that I were back on holiday. I needn't have worried though, Stafford wasn't bad at all, there wasn't much bathing, or shaving to do, and the bed making I could cope with, as it seemed to be the only physical work that I was called upon to perform I never had cause to wear my white coat on this ward.

As I entered the door I was met by Adam, he was a man, I later found out who had been a scientist, but he'd had a stroke and as was often the case it had changed his personality. He was swearing and cursing as I closed the door behind me, and if I hadn't have had the previous experience of Salisbury behind me I think I might have turned tail and run for my life. He was really threatening. Fortunately for me a young nursing assistant came to my rescue, and distracting him, allowed me to make my way to the office.

The handover was in full swing, but because of the surprise welcome that I had just received from Adam, I went straight into the office without thinking, even though it was forbidden.

"I see that you've met our star patient," the charge nurse Gerry was smiling as he broke away from the conversation he was having with his opposite number and the staff nurses from either shifts.

"Come in and sit down, as you're in the office."

He beckoned to an empty seat and introducing himself and the others and made me feel really at home. I was so embarrassed, this wasn't how it was supposed to be, and not qualified I shouldn't have been in the office at handover. As it happened though, I needn't have worried, because Gerry was probably the most laid-back charge nurse in the hospital, well at least most of the time.

Following the handover, which, though I didn't know who the patients were I found the proceedings extremely interesting, we all went outside to one of the tables lining the right hand side of the wide corridor and sat down for a cup of tea. I was introduced to Sue who was the large, cheery young nursing assistant who had come to my aid a few minutes earlier. There was the staff nurse, John who was likewise a cheerful and friendly chap, he was in his late forties and had worked there he told me, since he was a teenager. He had spent most of his working life as a nursing assistant until Gerry, with whom he obviously got on very well persuaded him that he ought to do his training. After he had qualified Gerry then cajoled the nursing officer into staffing him alongside of himself, they made a marvellous team.

Gerry seemed to spend much of his time in the office, while John looked after things out on the ward. Ken, who was the other nursing assistant, and who would stand for no nonsense from some of the more demanding patients was given the task of showing me around the ward and explaining its function.

"Any time that you want to come into the office and look through the patients notes, just feel free, as long as there isn't a doctors round going on." Gerry told me.

"You'll never learn unless you find out all about them."

Then he gave me a little warning.

"If a nursing officer comes in, for goodness sake look busy," he said.

'I think I'm going to like it here,' I thought to myself as I got up from the table to follow Ken.

The ward was wide and long with tables down one side and a large alcove where there were easy chairs and sofas, with a TV in the corner. There were no restrictions as to when it should be viewed, and the atmosphere was altogether more relaxed than Salisbury. Along the other side of this huge 'corridor' there was the clinic, food store and a couple of other small rooms used as storerooms.

Apart from these and a small consulting room all the others were what were called side rooms. Each of these had little windows in so that the nurses could shine their torches through at night to check that the patients were alive and well. They also had locks on and were sometimes used as seclusion rooms, although they weren't often used for this purpose if at all possible, as Gerry tried to control the patient's behaviour more by using reason, than by using other more draconian methods. Not that he had a lot to do with the patients, because as there were a number of doctors rounds during the week he was often confined to the office with them, or doing the paperwork that resulted from their visits. Actually he encouraged me to do quite a lot of the administration with him, this was great as far as I was concerned because I was keen to be involved and to gain as much experience as possible.

Beyond the day area and behind a frosted glass partition was the dormitory, along with a number of other side rooms. The patients coveted these, as they were away from the bustle of the ward and gave a degree of privacy.

There were the usual bathrooms, of course, and the ward being on the first floor gave a lovely view of the hospital grounds. The windows of the ward as in most others only opened a few inches to prevent people from either throwing themselves out, or absconding. This was particularly necessary on the acute wards where quite a few of the patients were under a section of the Mental Health Act, some even being admitted under home office restrictions, while they were undergoing assessment; due to their committing some crime, or because of antisocial activity.

As we walked through the dorm Ken approached one of the beds that had someone sleeping in it.

"Come on Phil, time to get up, you don't want to be sleeping at this time of the day." He said in a voice loud enough to create a grunted response.

"All right, in a minute," the patient said as he turned over.

We walked on and Ken asked me how I liked nursing, the usual thing, I found as people opened up a conversation on first meeting me.

"I like it, but it isn't what I expected," I replied, and then went on to tell him about the advertising literature.

"They wouldn't get many people to work here if they told the truth in those brochures," he laughed,

"But there's one thing for sure you'll enjoy this ward, true there aren't many of the type of patients that your looking for, but there are a few. Mostly, though you'll get a lot of valuable experience. Gerry isn't always the easiest of people, he can have a bit of a temper on him sometimes, but I wouldn't work with anyone else by choice. To my mind its one of the best wards in the hospital and I should know, I've worked on most of them."

We walked back towards the dayroom and as we did I was just thinking of how bright and clean everything looked in comparison to my last ward when we passed Phil's bed again.

"I'll give you two minutes to get out of bed Phil, or if not I'll drag you out," Ken said in a voice that was friendly, but serious at the same time.

A young lad in his teens immediately jumped out of bed, fully clothed and protesting, he strode off towards the dayroom.

"You've got to be firm with the young ones, or some of them stay in bed all day, especially the likes of that one," Ken explained to me.

The lad who had been sleeping was quite a nice lad I thought as I encountered him later that day. We got chatting to each other, and it was refreshing to be able to hold an intelligent conversation with a patient at last.

"My mother died of cancer two years ago," he told me and dad got married again just recently."

As a result he said he had felt pushed out and began hanging around with the wrong type of crowd. He'd started taking drugs and although at first it was only smoking the odd joint, he had in the last few months dabbled with more serious stuff. Although he was sure that he wasn't totally hooked, he had gone a little too far one weekend and had ended up unconscious in a friends flat. His friend being worried that he himself would get into trouble dragged him out of the flat and around the corner into an alleyway, then dialled 999. That, he told me was how he eventually ended up on Stafford ward.

After this conversation I went into the office for something and told Gerry briefly what Phil had told me and said how sad I thought it was, and how I felt sure that he'd learned his lesson.

"I think it's a good time for us to have a little chat about the reality of psychiatric nursing," he said as he invited me to sit down.

"The thing about drug abusers and people with a drink problem is that they can't be trusted, not that some of them aren't nice people, but most of them can't come to terms with what they are. Take, for instance young Phil, he seems a good lad and sounds plausible, but he isn't everything he seems. This lad comes from a nice family, but his uncle is a drug dealer and they used to go fishing together a lot when Phil was younger. That's when Phil started 'smoking,' but it didn't stop there, since the age of fourteen he's been on the hard stuff and his family have disowned him. The rest is true, he was in friends flat and they had bought some bad heroin, that's why he ended up in that state. If you want any visible evidence of what I've told you take a look at his arms."

I was shocked and embarrassed by this, but in the future I learned to check what was written in the patient's dossier before taking every thing that I was told to heart.

At around five o clock some of the patients who had been working in the hospital gardens, or at the industrial therapy unit came back onto the ward, among them was Noel, he had been a patient there for sometime and was one of the frequent admissions due to a long-standing illness, his diagnosis was schizophrenia. Noel was a quiet man who kept himself to himself, content to sit alone smoking, or wandering around the ward, looking at nothing in particular, his expression rather vacant.

I discovered that he was the father of Ronald who had been my assistant when I managed the boutique several years ago. I told him that I knew his son, but smiling a sort of half smile he didn't seem particularly interested.

Theirs was rather a tragic family, on the day that Noel had married Carol, her sister had been driving to the wedding, when she was involved in a car crash and was killed outright. Not a good start to married life, but things got worse, Noel after some time began to have mood swings, sometimes he was depressed and not speaking for days on end and at other times he became aggressive, even to the point of being physically abusive to Carol and their two boys. I had met Carol on a number of occasions and found her to be a rather attractive, but nervous, highly-strung woman in her early forties. She spoke very quickly and hardly stopped for breath, but she was absolutely loyal to, and defensive of Noel, even despite the fact that he was now, what was known as a chronic schizophrenic. Things in that area would only get worse and now Noel was spending more and more time in hospital.

Ronald, I remember didn't understand his dad, and certainly didn't accept that his past behaviour was down to his mental state. He would constantly badger his mother to leave Noel in the hospital and divorce him. Carol wouldn't do that though and had him at home as often as she could. His behaviour had now modified due to his medication, but still he needed frequent admissions, because, as was often the case with a psychotic illness when he felt better, he would stop taking his tablets. After a few days of non-compliance (as it was termed) with the anti psychotic drugs, he would become irritable and threatening, and Ronald, who still lived at home, would insist that Carol arranged for another admission. On top of all that Ronald's younger brother Timothy was terribly affected by it all and was disruptive at school, his behaviour towards his mother was hostile too, she wasn't able to instil any discipline into him, and in the end the school arranged for a psychologist to see him.

I felt really sorry for the family and especially for Ronald whom I had got to know really well. Even before I ever considered nursing as a career and before I met Noel, when Ronald told me all that was going on at home, and how he hated his dad, I tried to persuade him to be kinder in his heart towards him,

"Why can't you try and be a bit more patient with him?" I had asked, "It's not really his fault, he's obviously ill."

Quite rightly he told me that I hadn't had to live with it day after day, not knowing what sort of reaction he would get from his dad at any given moment; he felt that his mother was wasting her life and was like a doormat to her husband.

It was a great pity, as apart from this Ronald was a nice lad, who absolutely loved David Bowie,

Unfortunately for him he looked like David Cassidy, (they were two pop stars, by the way.) he would hate it when girls would come into the shop and get starry eyed over him, comparing him to David Cassidy, who he couldn't stand! The last time I saw Ronald he had become a Jehovah's Witness, I didn't like to ask him whether or not his conversion had changed his feelings towards his dad.

That same evening I was having a chat with one of the patients who I have to admit, seemed to me at the time to be a very strange individual. As we talked another patient came towards us and joined in with the conversation. Now I'm not making this up, though it does sound incredible I know! During the conversation one of them claimed that he was a prominent biblical personality, the other was quite taken aback by this.

"Well, that amazing," he said, in astonishment, " So am I!"

He went on to tell us that he truly believed he was also a well-known, though different biblical figure. I could hardly believe my ears; I had never come across anything like it in my life. One of them sported a long shaggy beard and certainly looked the part. The other was from a well to do family and spoke with an educated accent and if I didn't know better I could well have believed his claim. This latter patient was named Jonathan Wells-Browning and as he walked he leant backwards to the point that he appeared to be in danger of toppling over and when he put one leg in front of the other he moved slowly and deliberately, lifting his knee high into the air. It was like something off Monty pythons flying circus' ministry for funny walks. The staff in fact universally called it the 'Wells-Browning walk,' I know that it sounds like I'm mocking him, but I'm not really, I was very fond of him, as he was a patient who I came across many times in my early years as a nurse and always got on well with him.

Before I left for home that evening, after all the work was done it was quiet on the ward, some of the patients had gone to bed early, others were watching TV, but I noticed a man who sat at one of the tables with his face in his hands. I didn't know anything about him and decided to sit down next to him at the table. He told me that he was a teacher and he had been admitted for depression a few days earlier because He'd tried to commit suicide with sleeping tablets. His wife of twenty years had left him for another man. When the children had left school she had wanted to go out to work and have a bit of money to spend on herself. He didn't mind that at all, in fact, he told me, he had encouraged it; unfortunately she had fallen for the boss and had left home.

How often I, as a nurse was to hear similar stories over the years and how often I would feel useless in those situations.

I mean, how do you tell someone like that, that everything will turn out all right; the love of their life has gone and left them, there aren't any pills that'll fix that. There aren't any words that don't sound like platitudes in such circumstances.

From that day I would slowly come to the conclusion that I wasn't going to fix everybody's problems, and that the park bench on the advertising literature was an illusion, an ideal that I wasn't going to realise. That particular patient, by the way went home on leave after a few weeks, but died of a heart attack while he was away.

It was a nice day, that first day on my new ward, but it was a sad day too. Not just because of that last patient I had spoken with, but also because of all those I had had the chance to have conversations with that afternoon. Whatever had brought them there, all of them had a need and I felt, as I was to feel hundreds of times in the future, that I was inadequate for the task of fulfilling their needs.

Chapter 13.

I really liked working on Stafford there was so much going on. For instance, one day a consultant, Dr. Hartley came onto the ward and had a patient that he wanted to do deep narcosis on. This was where a patient was given an intra-venous injection of a tranquilliser; not enough to knock him out, but sufficient to make him so relaxed that he would, theoretically at least tell the doctor the truth to any questions that he asked. The process took place and I was allowed to witness it. Whether or not Doctor Hartley got the results that he wanted I don't know, but I found it interesting.

'I bet no one else in my group has been able to see anything like this,' I thought, and I felt really smug.

The doctor told me afterwards that hypnotherapy had been all the rage a few years beforehand,

"But," he said, with a big grin on his face, "I never did do it. I would have felt such a fool if the patient wasn't really under, and suddenly sat bolt upright and started to laugh at me."

This man was always my favourite doctor. I had a lot to do with him over the years and once visited his home, where every wall was lined with books. I could never really call him a friend, but he was the only doctor that didn't make me feel that I was inferior just because I was a nurse and he was one of the medical staff.

I spent a lot of time in the office while based on the ward, doing nursing notes at the insistence of Gerry, who felt that it would benefit me. There was only one pink sheet to fill in daily then; no care plans, no assessments, no named nurses, it was all so simple, unlike today.

One day when I was doing my office work, Gerry talked to me about his wife who was a lot younger than him. As he was telling me about her, he made quite a few suggestive remarks about the benefit of having a younger partner.

"I'm not too thrilled that she hates classical music, though, that's a real downside to things, I have to sit and listen to it with a set of headphones on when I want to hear the music." he told me.

"Still, she's a good cook, and of course a younger woman has other attributes, if you know what I mean." He winked at me as he spoke.

While we talked the telephone kept on ringing, interrupting our conversation and several of the patients came to the door, one after another, mostly for their cigarettes. I could see Gerry getting more and more irritated, until finally another patient came in wanting something. Gerry exploded and using language that I cant print, he told him in no uncertain terms to get out. A moment later the domestic supervisor wanted to ask him something. This was no problem because he fancied her like mad. As she was leaving Gerry dashed behind the door and made an unpleasant gesture just as the phone started ringing again.

"Busy little ward, isn't it?" Gerry remarked.

As I was nearest to the phone I lifted it up, but because of what had gone on in the last few minutes, and especially because of that last remark I couldn't say anything, I just exploded into hysterics. The pain from the laughter was so bad that I had to kneel on the floor, clutching my stomach, phone in hand, the person on the other end was the nursing officer and he wasn't very happy. In a silent agony I held the phone out towards Gerry who thankfully rescued the situation. I never got any flack from that incident, but I made myself scarce the next few times the nursing officer visited.

Although the doors to the ward were locked at times, they weren't always, it depended on the type of patient that we had in at any one time. Sometimes rather than lock it, we would take it in turns sitting by the door and monitor the patients, letting those who we felt could go out have their liberty, but preventing others, section patients, or potentially suicide's from leaving. We counted everyone on a checklist at the beginning of every shift and again before we handed the shift over.

John, the staff nurse would let me do medication with him and also help with the ordering of medicines once a week, so I was able to learn the names and the functions of the different drugs, as well as the side effects.

One afternoon after leaving the clinic room, I noticed a young lad who seemed to be behaving strangely. His head was turned to one side and he appeared to be trying to say something, but couldn't get the words out.

"What's the problem?" I asked, concerned and unsure of what was going on with him.

Unable to understand his reply I called for John, who in turn called for the doctor. When he arrived they took him into a side room and gave him an injection, after a while the lad came out of the room and looked as if nothing had happened. John told me afterwards that he'd been suffering from a condition called torticollis, a side effect of the medication that he was taking. Quite a few of the patients seemed to have a tremor because of their medication, another drug was given them to try and prevent this, but it didn't always seem to be successful.

A new admission arrived on the ward one day; we had been warned that he was coming. He was coming care of the police and we were told that he was very violent. One of the side rooms was cleared out so that we could put him into seclusion, and the 'heavy gang,' some of the toughest nurses in the hospital were called over to help out. When he arrived he was handcuffed and surrounded by around six policemen. Gerry went up to speak to him and asked him if he would behave himself if the handcuffs were removed. On receiving his assurance that he would, the policemen released him and left. After a while, seeing that there was going to be no trouble, the heavies left us to it. The new arrival was as compliant as a lamb and never gave us any trouble for the time that he was with us. Many times I've seen the same thing, it was as if they realised that we weren't a threat, and however violent they were on the outside, on the whole the 'violent' admissions were absolutely fine on our wards.

There was one patient on the ward of twenty odd patients that most people steered clear of. Dennis was a paranoid schizophrenic and was unpredictable. Even those that he hung around with knew that if he was hearing 'the voices' it was best to keep away from him. One day he turned his hostility towards me, not that I had upset him in any way, just that he had been 'told' that I was out to get him and that he ought to finish me off before I got in first. Without warning one evening he came for me, shouting and in a fighting mood. Fortunately, the other staff and one or two patients as well, caught hold of him before he could reach me. I was in fear of my life and didn't know what to do.

"Get into the office out of the way, and ring for help, pronto!" Ken shouted, as several of them held him down.

I didn't need telling twice, and a few minutes later a load of heavies burst in to help. Dennis was given an injection in the dormitory and order was soon restored. The next day everything was back to normal, if a little uneasy. A couple of days later when I no longer felt his eyes burning in the back of my neck and he had settled down to his normal self he apologised,

“I’m sorry, it was the voices, telling me to get you before you got me” he said, obviously feeling remorse.

I never felt safe with him again though, and was glad when he was transferred to a long stay ward a week or two later. I was really upset by the attack

“Why me?” I asked Gerry.

“No reason, its just the voices, it could have been anyone, but that lad is dangerous and one day someone’s going to get really hurt,” came the reply.

Looking through his notes I realised I hadn’t been the first, which gave me some comfort.

It wasn’t until many years later that I really understood what the voices really were. I had imagined that they were something that the patients heard in their imagination, though they were still very real to them. One day I was talking to a girl who persistently cut herself on her wrists and arms, she’d also swallow things such as batteries, because the voices told her to. She explained that the voices that told her to do these things were audible, as if I were speaking to her. She felt a real evil presence with her as if someone was in the room and she was afraid that if she didn’t obey then there would be some punishment. Of course there were those who cut themselves because it gave them some sort of real release from tension, but in this girls case it was the voices ‘making’ her do it.

I got myself into real bother during one shift. I was asked to take a patient down to the coach station and make sure that he got onto the coach to go on leave to his mum’s house, about fifty miles away.

“Don’t let him out of your sight, or he’ll clear off,” were Gerry’s firm instructions.

Everything went on ok. on the way down to the town, but while we were waiting for the coach to arrive, Peter decided that he wanted the toilet.

“Ok. But don’t be long,” I said and followed him into the toilets, standing outside of the cubicle while he went to do his business. After waiting a few minutes and getting worried in case he missed his coach, I knocked on the door.

“Come on Peter, you’ll miss your bus.” I said to the toilet door.

No reply!

I knocked again.

Silence!

To cut a long story short, he had escaped through a little window above the toilet and was nowhere to be found.

I went back to the ward absolutely worried sick about where he had gone to and also because I had made a big mistake and would be in trouble. When I got there, I entered the ward sheepishly and told Gerry. He was to say the least put out, and I was in the doghouse.

A couple of hours later the patient was brought back by two policemen. Apparently he had made his way back towards the hospital, but before he got there he decided to call at a nearby house. When the door was opened by an elderly lady he had pushed past her, saying that he felt tired and then proceeded to the nearest bed room, got into bed and went to sleep. No harm done, except to my reputation, I wasn't allowed to forget the incident in a hurry.

Forbes another patient that I met on the ward was a man in his thirties who had been ill for a long time with schizophrenia. He lived at home with his parents and was a nice quiet person, always polite and helpful around the ward, but he didn't really want to go home. We couldn't understand it because when his parents came to visit they seemed like really nice people, very concerned for their son. Well, one Friday evening his parents came to collect him, and off he went. That was the last we ever saw of him, he apparently went for a walk the next morning and walked straight into the river and carried on going until the water went over his head and the current carried him away. That really upset the ward for days afterwards, both staff and patients. Could anything have been done to prevent the tragedy? No one could answer that one.

There are a lot of other patients that I could talk about, but quite honestly there are far too many to go through them all, there is one though, that particularly sticks in my mind.

Norman was someone that I wanted to find time to talk with, but because he was so quiet and the ward had others more demanding, he seemed to be neglected a bit, he was quiet to the point of almost being mute and used to sit on his own in a corner out of the way of the rest of the patients. Admitted because he had been neglecting himself he was a middle aged man of about fifty and grossly underweight. One day I had nothing to do after the evening meal and medication were finished, so I sat down next to this silent man who didn't seem to enter into conversation with anyone at all.

"Norman," I started after a few futile moments of hoping that he would initiate things; I had brought him a coffee as an excuse for sitting next to him.

"Of all the people that I've had anything to do with since I've been here you are the one whom I can't fathom, I can't get to the bottom of you, can't make out what's going on inside your mind. What is it that's brought you here and why is it you always seem so low?"

He looked at me and didn't speak for a while. I started feeling a bit embarrassed, wishing I hadn't asked, as he stared into my face for what seemed like an eternity.

"It's cannabis mostly," he eventually answered slowly, almost stumbling over his words and certainly deliberating as he continued.

"The young people of today think it's clever to smoke dope, but I was smoking before most of them knew what it was, and certainly before the medical staff really knew there was any real harm in it. It's taken everything. I've no appetite for anything; for food, for family, for living. My wife has left me because I couldn't work, or even play with the children and I couldn't fulfil my role as a husband in the bedroom. I'm done for. That stuff has ruined my life, years I smoked it and thought it was good being one of the gang; and the smoking led to other drugs of course."

Again I didn't know what to say, nothing I could say, or the doctors could do was going to cure his problems. Without mentioning his name I used him as an example over the years, of how drug taking isn't worth it. Whenever I nursed any of these addicts that I frequently came across, not just in that hospital, but others I worked in I would tell them about Norman and people like him, but unfortunately most of them weren't really interested.

I was unhappy to leave Stafford; if I could I would have stayed, but I had to move on. I got a good report, not as good as the first one, on Devon, but almost!

The next two weeks as usual were spent in school, but there was a difference, we all had to take an intermediate exam at the end of it and if we failed our future would be in doubt. It took a while to find out the result, so when I went on to night duty, which was the usual thing as you moved into the second year, not only was I worried about that, but I had to face the thing that we were all dreading. Night duty; no one of the group was looking forward to it, and it made several of them physically ill. Nevertheless the next three months had to be faced, albeit through gritted teeth.

Chapter 14.

I admire anyone who has worked night shifts for any length of time, it's totally unnatural and plays havoc with the body clock. The children in the street playing and of course, screaming and shouting, the buses and cars whizzing past, not to mention the motorbikes, as I was trying to sleep in the daytime. I wonder who invented motorbikes, especially those that didn't have silencers?

Night work was a nightmare, (excuse the pun.) I got very little sleep over those weeks and I was, as a result grumpy and impatient with my wife and children. It seemed strange going to work when everybody else was getting ready for bed, but I didn't have a choice, it was part of the training. If I had have known about it from the outset I don't think I'd have signed up.

The ward I was assigned to was fortunately a geriatric one, small with only twelve patients. Because I was only a second year student I wasn't supposed to be on my own, but they were short staffed as usual, so they had a trained nurse on the adjoining ward who kept an eye on me. The ward had a door that opened onto his, so by keeping it open at night he was able to help me out if I was in difficulty, and vice versa.

This little ward was a nice place, with a number of single rooms that were in the form of a crescent at one end, and the main dormitory consisting of seven beds arranged in the main body of the room. The continent patients were all in the single rooms and so really, all I had to do was concern myself with the rest. 'Quite easy.' I thought, as I was shown round by the day staff before they went off duty. Actually it wasn't that simple at all; is anything?

The first thing I had to do was to give a cup of Horlicks, or hot chocolate to the few patients that were still up. Most of the others were in bed, at least all of the incontinent ones.

On the first night I was nervous and aware of the great responsibility that had been placed upon me, I was darting backwards and forwards between the dayroom, where the few were drinking their horlicks and the dormitory where the others were sleeping. I didn't want anyone to fall if they were to get out of bed. After a few nights I relaxed a lot and didn't concern myself too much, but on that first night I was in awe of the situation.

That night, after they'd finished their drink I helped those who needed assistance to get undressed and then I washed their cups up before finally closing the dayroom door for the night. It was strange being there, all alone, I knew the adjoining door was open, but I hadn't met Dave, the staff nurse on the other ward yet, he was obviously busy with his own workload.

All the patients were in bed by ten thirty and the place had fallen silent, apart from the odd snore, or someone coughing, and someone else maybe turning over in bed. I had a night light on a table next to where I sat, and I'd picked some old 'Time magazines' up from the dayroom, so I sat a while reading these. Within a few minutes Dave came through and interrupted me.

"Hi! You're Robert aren't you, pleased to meet you, I'm Dave, welcome to night duty."

He spoke so loudly that I wanted to tell him to be a bit quieter, because I thought he'd wake my patients up. He was though, a very nice chap and told me about the routine. Apparently there was an hour's break in the night where I could visit the kitchen and get myself something to eat. After I'd had my break then I would cover for Dave while he had his.

"No sleeping on duty, mind you. The nursing officer always comes around, and sometimes more than once a night, so be careful," he warned.

I took what he said to heart and I think I can honestly say that I never fell asleep, mostly because I was afraid of the consequences. It was hard though, especially when I'd eaten, and more especially between two and four in the morning, reputedly the time when most patients die in hospital, the body clock being at it's lowest. Oh the agony of trying to keep my eyelids from closing.

You could do what you like, go and get a cold drink, or walk around for ten minutes, maybe splash cold water on your face, but as soon as you sat down again, there it came, the enemy: drowsiness, worse perhaps than that was the twitchy legs. It was an agony, try as you will they wont stay still. You could swing them around, get up and have a stretch, but before you knew it they were at it again. For certain that's the torturous thing about working nights.

Of course there were the patients to distract me, and if my drowsiness, or twitchy legs got too bad I could, and often would do a 'round.'

A round consisted of putting a hand carefully under the bedclothes to see if the draw sheet was wet. There were no sheaths, or convenes to catch the urine in those days and to leave the bed nice and dry for the patients comfort and to the nurses relief. If the bed was wet I had to replace the draw sheet by rolling the patient towards me, pushing the wet sheet underneath him and placing another rolled up sheet against the patient, then dashing around the bed I'd roll the patient back towards me. If all went well I could whip the wet sheet out and tuck the dry one in on both sides, and the job was done.

There were problems sometimes though; if there wasn't a sheet between the patient's legs then the whole bed invariably would be flooded, I reluctantly called for Dave to help. The worse thing would have been if I woke someone up, and so I'd try and do everything as gently as possible. Nothing was worse than if a patient got up and started wandering aimlessly around the ward, not only would they probably awaken one or two of the others, but also they were often in danger of falling, or hurting themselves in some way.

Wanderers were sometimes placed in a Buxton chair, a seat that I've mentioned before; a chair with a little table screwed on in the front of it, which restricted movement, usually preventing the patient from getting out of it. It didn't always work with some of the more determined characters though, they would just wriggle their way out and my night duty would sometimes turn into a nightmare. It could be very difficult indeed trying to look after a wanderer, as well as doing the other jobs. It used to drive me wild some nights.

Dave was very good and would really go out of his way to make things easy for me and we used to have some really nice times together. He was a smoker and would often open an outside door to have a quick puff while the nursing officer wasn't around.

One night we were standing looking up at the sky,

"It's a full moon tomorrow," he murmured to himself, as he gazed at the sky. Then turning to me he warned “It’ll be a busy night tomorrow, so get a good sleep before you come on duty.”

“Why’s that?” I asked, not understanding what he meant.

“Well,” he continued drawing on his cigarette, “that’s why they used to call mentally ill folk lunatics years ago, didn’t you know?”

“I’ve never really thought about it, why should a full moon make any difference to anything?” I asked him.

Apparently, according to Dave, any night that there was a full moon was always busy; the patients were, for some reason more restless and difficult to nurse.

Sure enough the next night with a full moon was just as he’d predicted. The place was like Paddy’s market. Several of them refused to stay in bed and they were wandering through to Daves ward, who was already having the same problems, himself. In the end he came through to my clinic and gave out PRN. medication to some of the patients to help them settle. He explained that PRN. medication was discretionary, only to be given if the trained nurse thought it was absolutely necessary, and then, in the case of night sedation not after two o clock, or it would cause the patient to be drowsy the next day. Well it worked, the first part of the night was bedlam, but by about two o clock everything was bliss.

An epileptic patient who wore a helmet in the daytime had a fit one night. I'd been taught how to deal with a situation like this, but I'd never seen a grand mal seizure before and panicked when I heard him cry out. Instead of staying with him and ensuring his airway was clear and that he didn't fall out of bed, I went running through to Dave for help. He came rushing through and got me to stand on one side of the bed while he stood the other side and we observed him until the fit was over.

"Sorry," I said, ashamed of myself.

"Don't worry, it's pretty frightening the first time you see it, but you'll be better next time." He was reassuring.

The next time wasn't long in coming, and the next after that, because the patient went into a condition called status epilepticus; continuous fits, one after another.

"I'll call the doctor, or he'll never stop and could die." Dave told me as he left me to look after things.

In a while a doctor appeared and after a bit of discussion and deliberation, he asked Dave to draw up some Valium for an injection. Shortly afterwards the patient's condition improved and he slept for the rest of the night. I hoped and prayed that it wouldn't happen again while I was on duty, and fortunately my prayers were answered, as he was alright after that.

Funnily enough when I did an essay for my finals, Epilepsy was the subject that I chose and I received a good mark for the work.

I wasn't always on the one ward on night duty, sometimes the nursing officers would take it into their heads to send me elsewhere, why I don't know, except maybe to give me and the rest of the group more experience. One night I was asked to go to Salisbury, and the nursing officer made a point of telling me not to fall asleep, as he would be visiting sometime in the early hours.

It was pretty daunting having to stay upstairs on my own with fifty patients. By the time I got there it was late, as I was having to cover for someone who had gone sick and they had put a female nurse in my place on my normal ward.

Everyone was in bed and I sat alone in the midst of a load of snoring men all night, without anyone stirring, even to go to the toilet. I was a bit nervous, I could hear the odd creak from the floorboards and the windows rattling with the wind occasionally, but apart from that it was really quiet and a little scary. As it happens I didn't have a job keeping awake, because most of the night was spent in doing the odd check on the patients, torch in hand; or listening for the sound of the nursing officer coming up the stairs to pay me a visit.

He didn't come of course, why would he? It was wet and windy outside and he wouldn't want to come trailing across the grounds to see me, but he wanted to keep me on my toes, so he pretended that he would come around. In the morning I didn't know whether to be glad that he hadn't come, or to be mad that I hadn't had a break and hadn't been able to go to the kitchen to fetch something to eat.

On the subject of food, there was a marvellous kitchen at St. Andrews where some of the staff worked into the early hours to cater for the needs of the night staff. What lovely food they made. My mouth waters to think of the puddings in particular, even now.

Somehow I got friendly with the head night cook and she used to look after me as if I had been one of her own sons. The chips she served up were heavenly, I've always liked chips, but there was something special about those that Marg dished up. If heaven could be contained in just one of her little creations, then I was in paradise on a nightly basis. The puddings as I've already indicated were a delight. You name it Marg was there every night with something new and wonderful.

One of the best things was that because she took a shine to me, I got gigantic portions. This was just as well, because I was a bit short of money. In my first year I was able to get by all right as I had saved quite a bit while I was doing my last job, but now things were getting rather sticky financially. It wasn't just me of course, the other students were feeling the pinch, especially those who had families, but happily for all of us it was around this time that the government recognised that nurses needed to eat like the rest of the population and they gave us a big increase in salary. Not that it made a fantastic wage, but it did at least keep the wolf away from the door.

As I've said, I was assigned to other wards at times and one of those was a large upstairs, almost rambling place. It was so large that it was difficult to orientate oneself at night. During a few stints on this particular ward a patient went into a hyperglycaemic condition. He wasn't in a coma, but as I was checking the patients I happened to mention to the staff nurse that a particular patient seemed to be sweating a lot.

"Mind you it's warm tonight," I said unconcerned, really believing that nothing was wrong.

"Well spotted," came the reply, as the staff nurse rose from his seat to investigate.

It seems that the patient in question was a known diabetic and was slipping into a coma. My observation saved him from that, but the ironic thing was that I had no idea. I was sent downstairs to another ward for some glucose. The staircase I used was accessed through a door in the dormitory, it seemed particularly dirty and cold, but I was in such a rush that I didn't think anything of it.

After the crisis was over and the patient was better again, for some reason or other I told the nurse who I was working with that I had used that particular staircase.

"You shouldn't have gone that way," he said with a bit of a concerned look on his face.

"That staircase has been haunted for years, didn't you know?"

When I told him that I'd never heard of any ghost, he said to me,

"Didn't you notice how dirty it is in there? It's because none of the domestic staff will clean it; you see a long time ago a man hung himself in there."

To me it sounded like something out of a storybook, and I didn't really believe it at the time. Later on though I had to spend some time on the ward during the daytime, and one weekend just as a bit of fun, during my lunch break I went down the stairs and up again; only when I came up I was moving a lot faster than when I'd gone down. Certainly there seemed to be something strange about that staircase, or was it really because I had been told the story?

I kept my own council though, and when the next morning at handover the incident of the hypoglycaemic patient was discussed I had the happy experience of being the nurse of the moment.

One night I was staffed on another ward and was on duty with a staff nurse who was actually younger than me. He wasn't particularly interested in doing any work, and if a patient got up because they wanted a cigarette, he would tell them in no uncertain terms to get back to bed.

He spent the night studying form. He was into horse racing in a big way and had had enough of nursing, he felt the future was in backing horses. I have to admit, it was very interesting. He could tell me the names of various people that had done as he was doing and as a result had become millionaires. I don't know what happened to him, maybe he did become a millionaire, but there's one thing for sure, he didn't stay with us for very long.

That night, though he told me a story of a grey lady who wandered the ward at night, particularly, it seemed at that time of the year. He said that he knew of someone who had seen her float through the partition between the dormitory and the day room. Well, I was in my element. I didn't know whether or not ghosts existed, but if they did, then surely this was the place where they would be.

Of course nothing happened and I'm not really sure whether I was being conned, but there's one thing I know, there was no way that I was going to fall asleep on duty that night!

Another night I was on duty on Stafford ward with a retired nursing officer. When they were nearing retirement it was often profitable for a senior member of staff to drop a grade and work night duty, which paid considerably more in the way of wages. That way a lot of senior nurses enhanced their pensions, as the last two, or three years wages were used to calculate the pension, particularly if they worked night duty with the unsociable hours paid at a higher rate.

This nursing officer was off of the ward for some reason for a time. I did a round of the dormitory with a torch in my hand and I thought that I smelt something burning. I shone the torch in the area that I suspected the smell was coming from and eventually found the culprit. It was a pair of jeans, by the bed of a patient that, although he knew very well that he shouldn't be smoking in the dormitory, like so many others he had decided to do his own thing.

Smoking in bed was a common thing and the fire engine had to turn out several times a week to false alarms, costing the taxpayer a small fortune. With that in mind I got a bucket of water and put the offending pair of jeans into it. The fire was out, though in truth it was only smouldering anyway, and I thought that I had done a good job.

Not according to the ex nursing officer, though.

When he came back onto the ward and I told him what I had done he went ballistic.

"Don't you ever do anything like that again, Panton. The whole place could have burnt down if you hadn't have put the fire out properly. That's why we have policies, so you can follow them for everyone's safety, not ignore them, because you think you're cleverer than the rest of us."

I couldn't really see what the problem was, it had all turned out ok. In fact I felt more than a little peeved at his attitude, but in hindsight I realise that I should have called the fire brigade, because if I hadn't have put the fire out properly a lot of people could have lost their lives. At the time, though I couldn't really see his argument, I thought that I'd saved everybody a lot of money and effort.

It was around this time that I was obliged to move house because my lease was up, and I needed a night off because the removal date was in the middle of a run of night duties. I asked the nursing officer if it would be ok. if I had just one night off to see to things.

He said 'No, he couldn't spare me.'

Out of desperation I took a night off sick, I couldn't think of any way around the situation.

The night of my return the nursing officer visited the ward

"How did the move go, Mr. Panton?" he asked me nonchalantly.

"Well, thanks." I replied, feeling so embarrassed, because it was obvious that he knew what I'd been up to.

The worst thing that happened to me on nights was that a patient died and it was probably my fault.

I was on the ward that had the 'haunted staircase,' at one end of it. It was early in the night and some of the patients were still going to bed. The nurse, who was the ex nursing officer, was on duty with me, but he had left the ward for some reason and I was alone, making sure that everyone got into the right bed. Suddenly Dick shouted out, or rather I suppose, cried out in an agony. I rushed to his bed where he had collapsed as he was climbing into it and, saving him from falling I lifted his legs onto the bed. He looked awful, pale and sweaty, in the half-light. I could see that he was unresponsive, but to my great shame and remorse, instead of attempting heart massage (CPR.) on him, I panicked and ran for the telephone.

As usual when you want someone in an emergency it took an age to get hold of a doctor. When he did arrive, followed closely by the charge nurse, Dick was well and truly dead. I've never forgotten that night, or forgiven myself for not attempting resuscitation before phoning for help.

There was another man on my usual geriatric ward that would constantly wander around the ward crying out,

"Oh dear, oh dear. Help me, there's something wrong with me, I'm dying, please help me."

This went on for several weeks, with most of the staff putting him down as an attention seeker. However one morning he was found dead in bed, by the day staff.

I wasn't sad to leave night duty behind me, especially after some of the incidents I'd encountered. There would be other times that I had to endure it, but that first rotation was the most difficult, yet somehow the most educational.

I'm sure, that for all that most of the day staff thought of nights as being a backwater in nursing, I found it in some ways to be very rewarding and, lets face it, somebody has to do it.

By the way during my time on nights I learned that I had passed the intermediate exam, I was now officially a second year student.

Chapter 15.

After we had completed our night duty, we as a group, had to have another couple of weeks in training school. We were all relieved to have got this far and really got stuck in with our studies. We had a trip out one day to a secure hospital where some of the P.T.S. were somewhat interested in going to work after they'd finished their training. I personally didn't like it, with its high walls, locked doors on every ward and the nurses walking around jangling their keys. To me it seemed like a prison, even the cutlery had to be accounted for after every meal, so not left with patients.

When that study block was over we were all assigned as usual to our various wards, mine was Kent. A little bit like Stafford ward, it was laid out in similar way, with a long corridor leading to a dormitory area. This was slightly different though, because it had a small dormitory right at the very end of the ward that was used for ECT. For the uninitiated this is electro convulsive treatment.

ECT. has always been controversial, but to me at the time I didn't really know a lot about it. I was soon to become familiar with it though because three times a week in the morning I helped not only to prepare the beds for each session, but also to actively participate in the 'treatment.'

I wont go into the mechanics of it to any great degree, only to say that the patient usually had a course of six treatments over a period of three weeks, if the doctor deemed it necessary, then there could be a further course; most of the patients were willing to undergo it, some were more reluctant. Those on a section Twenty Six of the Mental Health Act didn't have any option, if the consultant thought it would benefit them, then they had to undergo it, like it or not.

I know that there are a lot of people that think the whole thing is barbaric, and certainly it seems that way, with the patient rendered unconscious by an injection, then another medication given to stop the breathing in order to relax them while they received a shock that causes a short seizure.

It doesn't sound too delightful, does it, but does it work? The answer to that is, sometimes but not always. I don't know what the success rate is, but I can think of at least one person who definitely improved after having ECT.

Maureen was a lady whom I nursed on an acute admission ward. She was around forty years old and her children had left school and found themselves jobs. I suppose she began to feel useless and at a loose end and sank into a deep depression. She was admitted in a neglected state. Not speaking to anyone and not eating, she would sit in a remote part of the ward and avoid any eye contact. Her husband was at his wits end, she wouldn't do anything, just sit there, he couldn't get her to wash, dress, or eat and in desperation he called the doctor who arranged for her immediate admission.

She was given ECT. at the earliest opportunity and after two treatments she was as bright as a button, helping out on the ward and chatting to the others, as if nothing had ever been wrong. Maybe everyone didn't benefit from the treatment, but when it was successful it made up, as far as I was concerned anyway, for the failures.

The charge nurse on Kent was a nice man, quiet and unassuming and pleasant to work with, He was about fifty, single and he lived with his mother. Unlike most of the other staff Ted didn't get involved in the social life of the hospital, and to all of us he was a bit of an enigma. Everyone liked him and he didn't have to ask twice if he wanted anything doing. People had a certain respect for Ted, and would go out of their way to make him happy. He didn't join in with the usual banter between the staff, though, and the only time I remember seeing him laugh was when one of the night nurses tripped up, and in the process of trying to prevent himself falling, hit his hand on a nail sticking out of the edge of a shelf. The air was blue with the language that resulted, and Ted was in hysterics.

There was a week while Ted was off on holiday and Michael; the staff nurse was in charge. He was, on the whole a good nurse, but that week he did something that I didn't agree with. In those days the seclusion policy was far more relaxed than it is today. I can't remember all of the regulations for it, but I do recall quite clearly that one of the patients was beginning to become quite disturbed and as a result, threatening towards the others. Ted thought he'd nip it in the bud, so several of us grabbed him and put him in a side room, so in Michael's words 'He could be taught a lesson.' The great problem with that was that it went on for several days.

Eric would bang on the door with his fists, and if that didn't work he tried kicking it. The only thing that resulted from that was that he got a few injections of a major tranquiliser. The few times that he was allowed out was to have a cigarette and that was very occasionally and two nurses had to be at his side at all times. This went on for several days and everyone was getting tired of it, but Michael wouldn't budge, he still felt that Eric hadn't learned enough respect.

One afternoon while Michael and the other staff were either in the dormitory, or busy elsewhere I was left in the dayroom on my own, apart from a couple of patients. Eric knocked on the small window in his door and gestured that he would like a smoke.

I told him "You'll have to wait, I'm on my own."

He put his hands together, pleading with me.

"Alright I'll give you one, if you promise me you'll behave." I told him.

He said he would, and I naively believed him and went to get a cigarette, thinking that he'd seemed more settled lately anyway. When I returned, cigarette in hand, I opened the door. Eric flew out and grabbed me by the throat, then rammed me against a wall, shouting and cursing. The patients sitting nearby came to my rescue and at the same time Michael and another nurse appeared through the dormitory door, wondering what all the noise was about. Eric was pulled off of me and he broke down crying.

"I'm sorry, really I am, but I'm going absolutely crazy in there, I've learned my lesson, please don't put me back," he pleaded.

He was put back into the room for a while, but after some discussion, was let out again a short time afterwards, with a warning that if he didn't behave himself he'd be straight back in there.

"And next time I'll throw the key away," Michael threatened. He wasn't smiling when he said it.

He wasn't smiling, either when he gave me a good dressing down for being so stupid. He did admit though that perhaps he'd let the situation go on too long, not that that excused what I had done, I felt for the rest of my time there that Michael didn't really rate me very highly.

From time to time on that particular ward we'd have an older nurse who'd retired and was working part time to supplement his pension. There was a feeling among some of the other staff that he wasn't really much use. He was looked upon as an old fogey who had no idea about modern views on psychiatric nursing; an old 'attendant.'

I actually liked Charlie, that older nurse, he knew what some of the others felt about him, but if he was upset by what they thought about him, he never showed it. I spent a lot of time with him listening as he talked about the past, and I found it fascinating. One of the stories he told me, was when one day I was looking at the fish swimming around in the tank that stood on a shelf in the dayroom.

"They used to have a budgie on this shelf, you know," he said with a smile on his face.

"It was here for years, until one day a Polish patient decided he felt hungry. He opened the door of the cage, put his hand inside, caught it and then bit its head off."

I could hardly believe it, but when I asked someone else they told me that it was quite true.

Charlie also told me of the time when a patient on his ward years ago tried to hang himself on his bed head, but the breaks weren't on the bed and as it moved along the floor the ligature that he had used snapped and he ended up sprawled on the floor, he didn't try it again.

There was also the night a patient died and Charlie and another nurse were designated to take the body to the mortuary. That day it had snowed very heavily, and during the evening the wind had made a snowdrift in front of the door they were going to use. As they opened the door the trolley sped down the ramp outside, the body slid off and disappeared into the snowdrift. They had to leave it there for the morning shift because they couldn't find it in the dark.

I don't suppose either of those last stories were completely true, but I found them exciting at the time, if a little macabre.

While on Kent ward I was hit by a patient, which was one of the few times in my career when I was actually injured. We had a man who was suffering from what was known in those days as Huntingdon's chorea. He suffered from jerky movements and had lost the power of speech. Looking back I'm surprised that he wasn't on a sick ward.

One morning I was shaving him, when all of a sudden I saw stars. When I came to my senses my nose was bleeding and I realised that he had thumped me. I don't know whether it was deliberate, or not, but I couldn't hold it against him of course, because he was so ill.

We had two or three 'characters' on the ward. One who had been admitted for a short time was a transvestite. I had never heard the term before and had definitely never seen a man dressed up as a woman before, except perhaps at a pantomime. I have to admit that I found it rather uncomfortable and training that taught me to be non judgemental was difficult to adhere to. Not that I would have been overtly disapproving, but I couldn't help feeling so inside.

As it happened he was a nice person, if a little colourful, and I grew to like him, warts and all!

The patient that I'd seen when I first wandered along the corridors looking for the place to get my uniform from, was on the ward too. He was someone who suffered from Parkinson's disease and he was difficult to have a conversation with, because his speech was slurred, but he went for his walks around the corridors on a daily basis and everyone knew old Victor. I have to be really honest and say I never really liked him. He would get really cross with me if I couldn't understand what he was saying to me, and I really tried to be kind to him, knowing that he couldn't help it, but you enjoy some patients more than others.

A sad admission we had was another cross dresser, a man who really wanted to be a woman, a nice person, effeminate, yet always pleasant. He told me of the torture he was going through, being in a man's body, but feeling like he ought to be a woman. He was treated for depression, but shortly after discharge he committed suicide.

Another person I liked although I cant remember much about him was Artie, he was from Italian-Irish descent and was the ringleader of a little group who liked to criticise the staff behind their backs and cause a little dissention on the ward. I liked him though and he always seemed to enjoy a chat with me. As soon as I came on duty he would call out

"Did she let you have it last night, Robert?"

A lot of the staff didn't like him and in the handover referred to him as the little weasel, but I have to admit that I had a soft spot for him.

One of the middle-aged female patients in the hospital would do anything he wanted for the price of a cigarette.

"When I worked in the hotel trade I could get anything I wanted from a girl," he'd complain.

"Now I have to pay for the services of an old woman."

One of his cronies was an ex marine who was brought in for some vague mental problem. He didn't seem mentally ill to me, in fact he spent most of his time chatting up the girls on the female wards and making appointments to meet them down near the cemetery. Why they called it the cemetery I don't know. I went to have a look one day and all I could see was one head stone. Anyway that's where Ross seemed to have his fun. He told me He'd say to them,

"I find you sexually attractive, do you want to come for a walk with me?"

It seemed to work, or at least so we were told. He was a nice lad despite everything and although he may not have been ill and he was certainly taking advantage of the girls that were in the other wards, I couldn't help but like him.

A student who was in a group higher than mine and was placed on the ward the same time as me was very disheartened by it all. It wasn't what he had expected and he wanted to leave nursing, but didn't know what he could do because he had no skills. He was about forty and had a wife and a young child and he didn't want them to suffer by him doing anything rash.

One day he came to me and whispered,

"What are you doing at lunch time?"

I was intrigued and told him I hadn't anything on.

"Well, I've found a way to make my fortune," he whispered, mysteriously.

It transpired that he'd bought a metal detector, but felt a bit foolish about it and so didn't want anyone else to know. We went out that lunchtime into the fields opposite the hospital, and for several lunchtimes at the weekends. I rather enjoyed having a go with the detector, but Richard got a bit downhearted at not finding anything. In the end we came to the conclusion we were just wasting our time, however in recent years several hoards of roman coins had been found by treasure hunters, but I think they must have discovered most of the buried treasure in our area before we arrived there. We never found a brass farthing in the area we searched. Richard found himself another job before long and left, a pity really because I enjoyed our little expeditions together.

We had one lad on the ward that was heavily into drugs, he would apparently even inject himself with other things other than heroin, just to see what effect he might get. He lay in bed most of the day and when he was up and about he wasn't very pleasant to the other patients, or the staff. One day I got a bit fed up with calling him to come and get his medication, and so being rather annoyed I tipped his mattress, not actually forcing him out of bed, but just trying to get him to co operate. He was really angry, but knew that if he were to go for me he'd end up in seclusion. He was discharged soon after, because the doctors could see that they weren't able to do anything for him.

A couple of years later I was taken on a tour of the nearby prison. The prison psychologist was an acquaintance of mine and he had arranged for several of the students to visit. It was everything that 'Porridge' portrayed it to be, with its cells all in a row, the passageways running around every level and the safety nets to catch anyone who might be tempted to jump. As we walked through the corridors who should I see but the lad who I'd annoyed when I was on Kent ward. He was walking in a file having a prison officer in front and another one behind. As soon as he caught sight of me he broke ranks and ran and flung himself at my feet, grabbing me around my ankles.

"Please, please get me out of here!" he pleaded.

One of the officers dragged him off and he went along with the others, I never saw him again. I'm quite glad about that though, as I was told afterwards that he was in there for attacking someone with a knife.

In a way I wasn't too sad to leave Kent ward and to get the next phase of my training over with. After the inevitable two weeks in study block we were all assigned to either the occupational therapy unit, or to some other equally 'exciting' department. I drew the short straw, the very boring industrial therapy unit.

I don't know whether any one who is reading this has ever worked in a factory, doing the same job day after day, until your brain feels that it has been destroyed. That was what it was like there, we were made to work alongside the patients, doing exactly what they did for three hundred, or so days of the year.

I know that it all served a purpose, and I also know that they received a wage of sorts, but I also couldn't help but feel sorry for them. If they weren't mentally ill before they started to work there, then one thing was sure, they could very well be seriously damaged after a couple of weeks interned in the ITU.

'Why did they do away with the farm?' I asked myself angrily. At least the animals would respond to them, and it needed a bit of brainpower to use the tractors and the combined harvesters. Even if they weren't allowed to use them there would be a hundred and one jobs that were worth doing and wouldn't dull the brain like this factory did.

Still, none of the students had a say in these things and we all got on with it knowing that soon we would move on to the next ward, unlike the poor patients.

Chapter 16.

Over the next eighteen months or so there were other wards and other departments to be contended with. The ward that I really liked and probably shouldn't have enjoyed so much was Cornwall, even though the other students told me that they thought it was boring. It was an extremely large and rambling place that covered two floors and was the home to fifty men. I say home, because that was what it was. Most of the patients had been there for many years and had formed friendships with each other.

The charge nurse, Donald on my shift was like a father to them. He had looked after them since the time of Noah, and they liked and respected him. He was sometimes a little like a sergeant major, bawling down one end of the ward to the other if he thought it was necessary, but he loved them all, and they loved him, as much as they could love anyone. All Donald wanted to do outside of his working hours was to tend his garden; he never ceased to talk about his radishes and his parsnips and he lived for his days off so as to spend time tending his flowers and vegetables. He retired a couple of years later, but didn't have long to tend to the garden, as he had a heart attack and died within a few months of leaving us.

It was Donald who taught me how to play snooker properly. I had played before as a lad, but had never quite got the grasp of it.

The wonderful thing about Cornwall was that it had its own snooker tables, not just one in fact, but two, and they were both full size.

The reason that most of the students didn't want to be placed on Cornwall was because nearly all of the patients went out to work during the week, either to the industrial therapy unit. or working in the gardens. To most it was the most boring ward in the hospital. To me, I'm ashamed to say, it was respite from the normal routine and it was an opportunity to learn how to play snooker really well. Mind you, it took a lot of practice to match Donald, after all he'd had years at it!

He used to say things like:

"Twice as many brains and you'd make a good half wit, Panton," if I missed an easy shot.

Sometimes when I made what I thought was a funny remark he'd say to a nearby patient,

"He thinks he's a wit, but he's only half right!"

He had a way with words did our Don!

Once he took me outside and pointed to a door near to the rear of the ward.

"Do you know what's in there, Robert?" he asked, knowing that I didn't have a clue.

"Well, I'll tell you," he said. "That's the old toilet blocks. When I first came here in the thirties we had to swill them out every morning, even if there was snow on the ground. We had to go back and forth with our buckets and, with the help of some of the patients we'd do what was without a doubt the filthiest job there was in the whole hospital. You lot today don't know you're born."

To me, he almost seemed to wish those days were back, so that the modern day students could go through what he had endured in his early days at the hospital.

Cornwall was perhaps the largest ward in St. Andrews, but because most of the patients were self-caring, there were usually only two staff on duty at any one time. During the week that left a lot of the shift for me to practice snooker!

I learnt absolutely nothing there, but enjoyed it nonetheless. The only time I remember it being a profitable experience was when a student spent a week with us and I was able to show her how to give injections. Because there were a lot of these to do every week, she was quite proficient at it when she left us, although she was scared stiff when she gave the first one and I had to almost force her into it. She became a very able ward sister some years later and I was pleased to have had some influence in her training, minor though it might have been.

We had one patient who didn't go out to work, this was Morgan, and he was rather a restless fellow and would wander up and down the ward most of the day. Usually he was quiet, but one day the domestics were in a small room that was used for storing some of the food kept on the ward. One of the staff was smoking.

Morgan came and told me. "You should tell him that he shouldn't smoke in there," he said to me.

He was agitated and obviously expected that I should do something about it in the absence of the charge nurse who had left the ward for a meeting.

"Do they usually smoke in there?" I asked, not knowing how to react, because I really felt that it wasn't my business.

"They do, but only because Donald wont do anything about it." Came the reply.

"If Donald thinks its ok. Then I don't see what I can do, really," I said. "After all its his ward, not mine."

I went to the room where the offender was smoking his cigarette and told him what Morgan had said.

"Oh, don't worry about him," Mike the smoker said, "He's always got a bee in his bonnet about something."

At that Morgan passed by the open door.

"You've got no guts," he sneered as he walked by, pretty obviously referring to me; his corpulent stomach sticking out in front of him as he spoke. A moment later he walked past the door again in the opposite direction almost spitting the words at me.

"You've got no guts."

Again and again he came by, and with words loaded with scorn he told me that I'd got no guts. I was getting quite perturbed by it all and when

Donald came back I asked him to have a word with him.

"The trouble is Robert, he's telling the truth," he told me frankly. "I'm just as guilty as anyone, I shouldn't allow it, but its easier to ignore the situation. Morgan won't say anything to me because he daren't. With you he doesn't feel intimidated, so he knows that he can get away with it, but you can't tell him off, because he's right really."

Those words of Morgan have haunted me down through the years, and if I ever take the coward's way out I can hear Morgan's voice saying to me,

"You've got no guts." Taunting me for my lack of courage.

One day Donald asked me to burn some old dossiers that had been found near to the incinerator and had obviously been missed by whoever had been given the job to destroy them.

"Mind that you burn all of them, they're not meant to be lying around for anyone to see." He said to me as I went to do the job.

I couldn't help but have a look inside some of them as I threw them into the flames. They were all from the turn of the century, and I confess that I was so intrigued by them that I kept one back and took it home. I still feel guilty about it, yet it is so interesting, even today, as the case of a man who had been sent to St. Andrews from the local prison in the late eighteen hundreds. He wasn't appropriate as a felon because he was suffering from delusions and even in those days it was recognized that he was mentally ill. There was even a photo of him looking truly mentally unwell. I still have that small dossier now, among my most treasured possessions.

On the odd occasion I was asked to work on the other shift with Jim, Donald's opposite number. He was a bit of a card, all he would do during the shift, would be to sit in the office and talk about the old days in Ireland, when he was a lad. Apart from giving out medicines and making sure that all of the patients were fed, he did nothing and was renowned for it throughout the hospital. Still he was interesting to listen to, as he talked about his 'mammy' and of the old days in Galway and other places he had been to before coming over to England to find work.

"Things were so bad at times that we could barely afford to eat," he would tell me.

He'd talk about the furrows still to be seen on the mountainsides in the West Country, where in the eighteen hundreds the potato harvest failed due to the blight. Many of the inhabitants of the villages and the small farms emigrated to America and elsewhere, or starved to death, he said.

In his own younger days thing weren't much better and the men would often come over to England and work at digging trenches, or other backbreaking jobs, just so they could earn enough money to send back to their families. Jim was one of the lucky ones and had landed a job as a nurse. It didn't pay very well in those days, but it was better than being out in all weathers doing manual labour.

I moved on from Cornwall ward to a nightmare. The charge nurse on my next ward was a keep fit fanatic, and would spend his evenings at home lifting heavy weights.

Another nurse who lived next door to him warned me

"Bernard's a nutter," he said, shaking his head, "He keeps my wife and I awake at nights with the sound of bump, bump, as he lets the weights drop onto the bedroom floor; the whole house shakes."

I don't suppose he was a 'nutter,' as such, but he was a strange man, nevertheless. Later on I would nurse his sister who was a chronic schizophrenic, and I did wonder that maybe something might have been shared in their genes!

When I first arrived on the ward he was friendly enough, and invited me to join him and the other staff for a cup of tea. He was drinking milk.

“It helps to keep the blood sugar up,” he explained.

“We all need to keep the old blood sugar up on this ward, don’t we lads?” He asked, looking around the table at the others.

They all agreed as one man, and I became a little disconcerted. What did he mean? To me by now, long stay wards, though different had pretty much the same type of work and I couldn’t see this being a problem.

“You need to be physical to work here, lets have a look at your biceps,” he demanded good humouredly, rolling up the sleeve on his own white coat so that I could admire his well developed muscles. I obliged, feeling extremely self-conscious of my puny example. There was a loud burst of laughter from the others, naturally.

I wouldn’t have minded any of this if it had stopped there, but every tea break he would go on in the same vein and the others would laugh and agree obligingly as if all this were normal conversation. He would try and get me to drink milk instead of tea.

“After all you need to keep the old blood sugar up.” He would repeat over and over again.

I was beginning to get a bit bored by it all and didn’t like the same old drivel day after day. On top of that he wouldn’t let me do my job.

If I were in the bathroom he'd come in and start to show me a 'better method' of cutting toenails, or washing a patients hair, etc. In the dayroom he'd get me throwing a ball to a group of patients and then join in so it was done in the correct manner, which really irritated me.

At home I felt depressed and was short tempered, until Bev suggested that it was time I found another job.

"I can't stand you coming home in a bad mood much longer. If you're not happy get out, there must be better ways of earning a living and with a lot more money, as well." She told me one night after I'd bitten her head off over something really trivial.

After about three, or four weeks of it I couldn't stand any more I and went to see Rees.

"I'm sorry, but I can't work on there any longer," I told him, and in desperation said that he'd have to arrange a move for me, or I'd leave.

Rees was non-plussed, no one was ever moved during a placement, and the nursing school wouldn't normally give in to any request by a student if they had a preference for a particular ward.

"Ok. Robert, I can see that you're upset," he said, after pondering the situation for a few moments, "I'll see what I can do, but I don't hold out much hope."

I left his office and on my way home bought a newspaper to begin looking for another job. The next day I arrived on the ward and was told that I was to go and finish my placement downstairs on a female ward, Rutland.

Bernard said nothing to me about the decision to move me, he was probably as embarrassed as I was, and therefore he was unusually quiet.

I went as I was told to my new ward, and was met by a really nice sister.

"Male students don't normally work on here," she said, "but I understand you've had a few problems." Lifting her eyes up to the ceiling and the ward upstairs, smiling a knowing smile as she spoke.

No more was said and I was shown around the ward and told that I'd not be able to do some of the more personal care with the female patients and would have to make myself useful by doing some of the none nursing care tasks, I gladly agreed.

It was nice working with the old ladies, there was hardly any swearing, or smoking and the atmosphere was happy and relaxed. The staff were friendly and kind to me, not seeming at all resentful that they were doing most of the heavier work.

I learned how to put the ladies stockings on, the type that went just above the knee. I also became quite adept at twisting the top of the stocking and tucking it in so that it wouldn't fall down as they walked around. They were mostly lovely and cheery.

One day I couldn't get one of the ladies arms into her dress and I said,

"Shocking Mrs. Cocking."

"Two legs in one stocking," the old lady finished off.

I had only known the first line and was thrilled that she had taught me the rest of that little ditty.

I used to take some of the ladies to the church services on a Sunday morning and to the ballroom during the week, where they would be able to pick new dresses for themselves from a lady who came in from time to time with a selection for them.

One of the patients had a sore on her heel that had become a bit of a problem, so several times a week I'd take her down to the physiotherapy department so she could get ultra violet treatment on it. Amazingly the sore got better after a few weeks and she was back to normal.

Nothing lasted forever and I had to move on in a few weeks, but I shall never forget those ladies and the way they were lovingly looked after by the staff on Rutland ward.

After that some of the PTS were obliged to do two weeks up at the general hospital. Few of us liked it, as we felt that being the first set of psychiatric students that had been placed there we were rather in the way of the extreme busyness of a general hospital.

I ended up on casualty for a week of my time there and I hated it. The sister, who was a woman in her late forties, was a bit of a taskmaster. She would get me to dust the department, and then go around the curtain rails and other out of the way places with her fingers and give me a dressing down if she found any dust. She always did, without fail, and made a point of it. Some days she would wear a wedding ring and others not; one of the auxiliaries told me that she had a boyfriend and if she were seeing him that day, then she wouldn't wear the ring.

I wasn't able to do anything in the way of nursing care while I was there, as I was only there to observe. Unfortunately, (or fortunately) it was a quiet week and there were only two people that I remember being brought in by ambulance. One was a man who'd got his head stuck in a revolving door and had to have a large piece of his scalp sewn back on again. The other was a nurse from St. Andrews who, while on the way home from work had fallen off her bike and needed some minor dressings.

The second week I was assigned to the children's ward. Funnily enough it was the one I'd been a patient on myself, as a child. It was nice to work with the children, most of who were in for just a few days and had had a minor operation. What I didn't like though were those who had serious illnesses and injuries. It was heartbreaking to hear them whimpering and calling out for help. The staff of course, were kind and gentle and couldn't do enough for their little patients. I was glad to leave the hospital after my two weeks, though and looked forward to getting back to what was for me by now, normality.

Chapter 17.

My next ward and the last one before I took my final exams was an acute admission ward. I had waited so long for it, but when it came along all the big ideas I'd had before I began my training were now a thing of the past. By now I had my feet firmly on the ground; if I could help someone in distress that would be wonderful, but I wasn't expecting to do miraculous things anymore.

Orchard house was a long single story building consisting of two-mixed sex wards, separated by a long corridor where the out-patients surgery was held during the day. I was staffed on the west wing, which was served by three consultants. To say it was busy would be an understatement. During the week each consultant had a ward round and they saw all of their patients. A couple of nurses and some social workers, along with any other interested parties would be present. One of the consultants had a lot of young drug addicts and personality disorders, most of who were in trouble with the police, so his case conferences, as they were called were elaborate affairs taking a lot of the day up, as well as requiring around ten to fifteen people to be present.

During each weekday there were a number of junior doctors who visited the ward and I was able to gain a good deal of experience by sitting in with them. At the weekend it was a lot quieter as many of the patients went home on weekend leave.

My first day on duty was a Sunday and one of the patients, who happened to be a GP wanted to go out for a walk. As I was new and useless as far as the ward routine was concerned I was asked to accompany him. I was told not to let him out of my sight as he was on a treatment section. He had an alcohol problem and before admission had chased his wife around the garden in a drunken rage, holding a carving knife in his hand at the time. The consultant was concerned that if he were to leave the hospital he might go back home and kill his wife.

This time I didn't make a mess of things and brought him back safe and sound, but not before I had had a very interesting walk with him.

James knew the names of all the trees in a wood at the edge of the grounds that we strolled through. I'd always liked going down to the woods near where I lived when a lad, but I'd never taken any notice of the many different types of trees there were. He didn't tell me anything about himself and I suspected that he rather resented my playing the part of a prison warder. Nevertheless he showed me the differences in the various types of leaves and the flowers as we passed and challenged me after a while to tell him which tree and flower was which. I had several of these walks with him over the weeks and got to know what was what in that area, but never got to know anything about him as a person.

Over the years I nursed James a lot, he was constantly in and out of the hospital that I would eventually work in when I became a charge nurse. Although I got on really well with him, he was a closed book. Strangely enough when he died five, or six years later, though he was a heavy drinker he didn't die from liver failure, but from cancer. He always boasted to me that he could control the damage to his liver by taking high doses of vitamin c.

As time progressed I was able to do the necessary assessment for the medication round, which consisted of being questioned on every medicine I gave out to the patients. I passed that and so then went on to having to set a trolley up for a catheterisation, and of course being questioned about it. Again I passed and was nearing the end of my time as a student.

During my time there, I made one of my many blunders. I was in the office one day when someone rang with an urgent message for the staff nurse, she was nowhere to be found, so I took the message and instead of writing it down, I memorised it. The only trouble was that the ward was so busy that I forgot to tell the staff nurse. She received another call later, but it was too late and the consequences could have been disastrous; she was livid with me.

"Don't you think you should have told me about that call, Robert?" she asked.

She didn't make a meal of it, but let me know in a very quiet way that she was furious. Up until then she had always thought highly of my abilities, after that she may not have been quite so sure.

While on that ward we had a man admitted, accompanied by several policemen. He was a very well built man. After the police left he paced up and down the ward like a caged tiger. When he saw that I was alone, as the other nurses were either off the ward, or in a doctors round, he came to the office.

"I'm leaving," he said. "Are you going to try and stop me?"

I felt my heart thumping at a lot more than it's usual rate. "No, but I think you ought to stay until you've discussed it with a doctor," I answered trying not to sound too afraid of him.

"Stuff the doctors!" he said in a most unfriendly manner.

Then he turned around and left the ward. It was a few moments before I worked out what I should do, I didn't want to look like a coward, but he was a very big man, so I reasoned with myself that I had done the right thing. Fortunately when I was able to tell the sister she agreed with me. The police caught him up with later and fortunately he wasn't brought back to Orchard house.

One of the patients on Orchard was a 'cutter', a surly girl of about my age. She would get a razor blade and make minor cuts on her wrists. She'd been in and out of hospital for years and many of the staff were a bit tired of her, feeling that they ought to be helping others that were 'really ill.'

Poor old Sandra, I don't suppose she could help it, but she was tiresome. The first time I saw her after one of her cutting episodes I was walking up the corridor towards the office. Sandra was standing outside with her arms dripping with blood and her face showing 'attitude.' I ran back to the TV. room and fetched the staff nurse. Normally Lisa was a very caring person, but when she saw the object of my panic she turned on her heels and walked back to the TV. Room.

"I'll see to her in a few minutes," she said, obviously irritated.

Later on she told me that the policy with Sandra was to ignore that type of behaviour initially, and to get her to clean her cuts up herself in the clinic room when the staff felt it was convenient. I couldn't agree with their policy then, or later when I came across it in other hospitals, but I wasn't in a position on Orchard to argue, so I conformed when it happened again in the future, which it inevitably did on numerous occasions.

My training as regards holding non-judgmental attitudes came in for some testing, when I found that we were nursing a young man who had shot his stepfather dead for the simple reason that he wasn't his real dad. He was a quiet lad and I never got into a conversation with him, I don't think anyone really got to know him well. He spent some years in the hospital, I understand, but no one was ever able to say he was 'cured' before his eventual discharge.

Then there was the teenager, a lad who looked like a young version of Tarzan. He had hit a girl over the head with an iron bar. I found it difficult to understand the reason why. These weren't the only ones on the ward of course, but as a sample it just gives an illustration of the type of patient that we had to deal with, all the time being impartial; it could be hard sometimes.

While I was there I had to take charge of the ward for one shift as part of my training. What a difficult time that was, how I prayed that nothing would go wrong. Happily I got through the ordeal and passed the assessment!

Towards the end of the three years I, and the others in my group had to undergo the final exam. We were all afraid, even the brainy ones and none more than myself who wasn't one of the brightest in the group. I had a cunning plan though. I had become friendly with a second year student who had a phenomenal memory. The day before my finals I arranged to be staffed on his ward so that I could pick his brains. It wasn't easy to sort this little arrangement out, and I'm sure that it wasn't easy either for my ‘mentor,’ with my following him around all day asking him questions; but it worked!

The next day as I sat down and opened my questionnaire I knew that I was going to pass. Nearly every question was on something I had gone through with Robin the day before. Of course I couldn’t be sure, but I was happier about that exam than I had been about any other since I had been a student. After the exam we all went for a drink in the social club and talked things over, some quietly optimistic and others down in the dumps.

Life went on though, we all had to return to our various wards and await the outcome of the exam. Not only this but, unfortunately we had to have an interview as well. If we passed the exam and were to become staff nurses then we had to have a job to go to and it was necessary to apply for one.

We all went along at our appointed times and everyone was successful, dependant of course on the outcome of the final exam, everyone except me that is. As usual I had made a bish of it! We were asked in the interview where we would prefer to work if we were successful. That shouldn’t have been a problem, except that I’d told the panel that I didn’t want to work on a geriatric ward.

I went back to orchard after the interview, congratulating myself that it had gone well; it hadn't! During the evening my nursing officer came onto the ward and ordered me into the office.

"What do you think you were doing Panton?" He fumed. "Saying that you don't want to work on a geriatric ward has lost you your job!"

"Now look here you stupid idiot," he continued in the same angry tone,

"I've arranged another interview for you. It's at nine o' clock in the morning. I don't care if you're on duty or off duty. You'll be there! And you'll tell them you'll work wherever they want you to work. Do you understand?"

"Yes," I answered, feeling really ashamed of myself and upset by his raging tirade.

"And thankyou," I mumbled, scarcely able to get the words out. "I'm sorry, I didn't think they would want people working where they're not happy."

"Don't think; just comply, will you?" He raised his hands in the air in exasperation, and murmuring a barely audible 'Goodnight,' left the office.

I went for the second interview, of course and ate humble pie to get the job, but the worst thing about it was that it was all over the hospital that I had messed up. Everybody knew and they were all sniggering; I was so embarrassed and it took quite a long time for people to forget.

Chapter 18.

I passed! I passed my finals!

It was one of the best days of my life, I had done it, and I was a staff nurse! It was a happy, sad day though.

I went to visit my father in law in hospital who was dying of cancer and told him. He had been waiting for the news and although he was under the influence of morphine and was confused he understood.

"Well done, I've waited for this day so long," he said in a semi delirious tone.

It was the last time I would see him. The rest of the family and all my friends were delighted for me and I myself could hardly believe it after all this time. I could now write a letter and put RMN (Registered Mental Nurse) after my name.

More or less as soon as the news was received at the hospital I was transferred to another ward. Not, as I had feared to a geriatric ward, but to the other wing of Orchard house, I was delighted! This was when the serious stuff started though; here was where I really began to learn about psychiatry. Before, my mistakes could be forgiven, now I had to pay the price for anything I did wrong.

Inevitably I did something that got me into trouble. It concerned a certain consultant that was supposed to do his ward round on a Tuesday morning at eleven o' clock. He was always late and the staff made allowances for him.

One morning I was in charge because the sister had a day off. The consultant was late, very late. He didn't turn up until twelve thirty and the patients were all eating their midday meal. I had waited and waited and held back the lunch as long as I felt I could, but as he still didn't arrive I served it up. Lo and behold, as soon as it was on the table he appeared; I was fuming.

"You'll have to come back later," I told him. "The patients have been waiting for hours and they're having their lunch now. Don't you think it would have been courtesy to telephone and tell me you were going to be late?" I asked.

Without saying a word he left.

The next time I came on duty I was met by a nursing officer who told me in no uncertain terms, that I couldn't treat consultants like that. To be fair the rest of the staff including the sister thought it was wonderful. They had wanted to do the same thing, but daren't. Little did I know that I would meet the same consultant in the future and we would, on the whole have a good relationship.

The sister on my new ward was wonderful, absolutely lovely. She really took me under her wing and taught me so much about running a ward. Sometimes I would be walking along the corridor that extended from one end of the ward to the other and she would be walking from the other end towards me, and I approaching her from the other end.

"Heathcliff!" she would cry.

"Kathy!" I called out in return, and we ran towards each other; then taking her in my arms I would swing her round, as if we were playing a part in Wuthering Heights, we enjoyed the joke. She was lovely to me, an insecure staff nurse, and I really appreciated her informality in what was often a very formal atmosphere. It was a great shame that she left after just a few weeks, due to the breakdown of her marriage. One thing that she taught me was to listen more and not to give opinions when speaking with distressed patients, something I had learned in school, but she was keen that I followed it through on her ward.

It was at this time that I learned of my former tutor Rees's death. He had told the PTS. during one of his lectures that he and his wife had problems, but they weren't too serious as far as he was concerned. Unfortunately he must have underestimated the situation and she obviously saw it differently as she ran off with someone else. Rees because he was so upset resigned his post and went to live with his mother in Wales. Within a few weeks he suffered a heart attack and died. Not only did he pass away, but also Paddy who had shown me around the hospital only just over three years before went the same way. I suppose that because there was so many staff working at the hospital it was inevitable that some of them would die, but it was sad for all of us who worked there.

I was devastated when Lynne, the sister resigned. She was such a lovely person that at first I didn't give the new sister a chance.

Pat was a good nurse, an Australian who had come over to England to find her roots. It took a few weeks for me to warm to her, but after a while I realised that she was a good and caring nurse. She was supportive to me when one of my cousins was admitted to the ward with depression. I found that very difficult. It was a situation that I hadn't bargained for, but Pat helped me through the situation. I was only allowed to speak to my cousin on a superficial basis, Pat was the one who got more deeply involved and after a few weeks he was discharged without my feeling that I had let him down in any way.

After a few months I noticed an advert in the internal mail. It was for the position of charge nurse at The Friary. The Friary was a small psychiatric hospital on the other side of town. There was something about it that I liked the look of, but several staff members warned me that to go there was to ruin my chances of advancing my career. Nevertheless I knew the hospital and I wanted to try for the job, despite my lack of experience.

When I was a lad one of my friends knew a patient in that hospital and we had visited him. I couldn't remember much about the details, but I felt that I would like it. After all I wasn't likely to get a senior post at St. Andrews after my track record. So I asked for an application form for the vacancy. When it arrived I filled it in and showed it to Pat.

"You are joking, aren't you?" was her reaction.

"If you send this in you'll definitely not get the job," she said emphatically.

She made me send for another form and then instructed me how to complete it: No negatives, only positives, and so I received an invitation to attend for an interview.

"Go in looking positive," Pat said.

She should have known, I thought, she was Australian and they were always so full of confidence.

I wasn't confident, far from it.

Entering the grounds of The Friary by the rear door. I walked through the gardens looking up at the huge pillars that stood before what was obviously the front door a hundred years ago. I then walked past the trees that were in abundance and recalled later one of the nurses telling me how she would come on duty in the morning, hearing the sound of the owls as they hooted in the dawn light. I went around to the front door and entered the reception area in fear and trepidation.

"Can I help you?" The girl in her little cubicle asked, with an unfriendly tone.

I told her who I was and why I was there and she asked me to wait until she could find someone to meet me. Thankfully that particular girl had just given in her notice and was to be replaced by someone else. I don't think I would have got on very well with her if she'd stayed.

I was nervous at the interview, and although I don't recall much of it, I felt sure I must have said various things that portrayed me up as being lacking in knowledge. The good thing was that one of the applicants hadn't turned up and the only other applicant was a woman who had applied before for a job and had been turned down. After the interview I was shown into a small room while the panel of one consultant and two nursing officers debated our performance. I thought that the other applicant was more nervous than me, but she was older and more experienced, so I didn't think I stood a chance.

After a few minutes the door opened and she was called in and I never saw her again; another few minutes passed, then I was asked to go into the office, feeling sure I was going to be turned down.

I wasn't. I had been successful, with a month's probationary period.

I could hardly believe it and was so excited that I feel now that I behaved in an overexcited way saying silly things in my relief at getting the job, and that the interview was over successfully. The panel forgave me though, and I was told I would start as soon as the managers could release me from St. Andrews.

I had walked to the interview, but I flew home as if I had wings, to tell everyone who would listen; I, Robert Panton who I myself believed to be one of the worse students in my PTS was a charge nurse after only passing my nursing exams ten months before. What had The Friary let themselves in for?

Chapter 19.

The Friary was so very different to St. Andrews that I felt uncomfortable there for a long time. Fortunately for me Jenny, the sister on the other shift looked after me and often covered for any mistakes, which were a little frequent, especially at first.

I visited Shackleton ward a week or so before I was due to start there as the new charge nurse opposite Jenny. No one liked her, she was a southerner and could be quite brittle, but towards me she was always kind and supportive, because I was young and new, and she must have realised I was almost out of my depth. She was like a guardian angel to me. No one could say a word against me, but she would jump to my defence. I was so lucky. She was a woman in her mid thirties and hated The Friary, but because her husband had a good job on the children's unit within the grounds of the hospital she unwillingly stayed.

On my visit I didn't notice the carpeted floor, or the abundance of antiques, I was too nervous. Later I realised what a beautiful place it was.

There were only five wards, four in the main block and then the children's unit, which stood some way from the main building. The Friary was a smallish red-bricked building that had been built in Georgian times and was at one time a private mental hospital. Now there were still private patients, but most of the beds were for NHS patients.

In the dining room, which was shared by Shackleton and Ross the other upstairs ward, there was an enormous portrait of one of the founders, and the whole place shouted history.

Apparently when the central heating system was put in, the workmen found a number of valuable rings under the floorboards that must have slipped between the cracks before the wards were carpeted.

Down in the cellars, which I explored at the weekends, when the nursing officer wasn't around, were two skeletons and jars of ancient organs in bottles lining the shelves, I imagine that it had been a teaching hospital sometime in the distant past.

There was another great difference between where I had worked before and this place, if any nursing staff in the area had a mental problem, they would invariably be admitted to The Friary. As a consequence I had the embarrassing task of looking after some of the staff I'd worked with previously. One in particular was a little difficult, but I treated her just the same as anyone else, she was a nurse who, in my childhood had owned the local sweetshop in my neighbourhood. The times she'd told me off for dithering in her shop, while I wondered which type of sweetie I should buy when a child; now she was a patient on my ward and in my care

I sometimes found it difficult during my time there, not least when the retired chief medical officer from St. Andrews was admitted with depression. I found it difficult to deal with him, and to be honest tried to keep a bit of a distance. I don't think the consultant in charge of him liked it much either, because he had worked as a junior under him years before. I'm afraid the situation didn't work out very well, and sadly this patient went on weekend leave and committed suicide by putting a hose onto his car exhaust and killing himself with carbon monoxide gas.

The visit I made to the ward, to get an idea of what was expected of me wasn't inspiring. I got on well with Jenny from the start but she admitted that she knew she wasn't well liked. We made a pact that if anyone should say anything disparaging about either of us, the other one would say only nice things in return. I was to be faced with this problem on my first day, both from staff and patients, as Jenny was really unpopular, but I tried to never allow this gossip when I was around.

She introduced me to some of the patients when I was familiarising myself to the ward. There were four who had been there for very many years, despite it being an acute admission ward, which meant that the stay should have been for less than three months.

One of these was Minnie, who was a woman in her fifties, with shoulder length grey, unkempt hair. She spoke with an upper class accent and in her previous life had been a ladies companion, travelling throughout Europe. She believed that a prominent member of the European royalty was coming to marry her and whisk her off to his palace any day. The trouble was that she had been waiting over twenty years for him to arrive.

Minnie was a highly intelligent woman with a fixed delusion and her consultant was so taken with her, he used to bring his medical students around to interview her at times. She wasn't at all concerned by this and was glad to be able to talk about her Prince. She would often write to him and speak of her love for him and her impatience at the length of time he was taking to fetch her to her new home. The hospital received several letters from this Prince about the situation and when things were explained to him, he said that he was happy to keep on receiving the letters if it was therapeutic for Minnie.

She didn't like me very much on sight. Not because I said anything wrong, but because she felt that I was rather common and also she had loved the sister the place of whom I had taken. This was often a common feeling with the patients, apparently, whenever there was a change of staff.

"Oh, you would have loved her, Mr. Panton, she was so refined and spoke beautifully, it's such a sad loss," she said.

Minnie sat with her legs crossed, one foot swinging to and fro as she puffed away at a cigarette. She coughed every time she inhaled.

"Why don't you give up smoking?" I suggested.

"It's my only pleasure," she spluttered "I've been incarcerated in this place for so long, I have to have something to distract me; but my time will come." She told me confidently.

Dear old Nigel, another of the long-term patients had been there forever and his only activity was to study. He'd been at Cambridge and had graduated with honours, but because of a breakdown associated with his studies he'd landed up at The Friary. His abiding passions were to study for several hours of the day, for no particular purpose, and also to sit in a chair that overlooked the ancient church that could be seen from out of the window opposite. Woe betide anyone bold enough to seat themselves in his place, he may have been a gentleman normally, but he knew how to use swear words, if he felt it necessary.

It was during this transition that I learned that the cleaners were called ward maids and I was known not as a charge nurse, but as 'sister.' I soon put a stop to that!

Shackleton was made up of two long corridors, with single rooms coming off at intervals and a large female dormitory, as well as a few double rooms and another smaller dorm. It was huge, with a large sitting room containing a grand piano and a hairdressing room, as well as a library used by all of the hospital patients and also a large occupational therapy area next door. It had everything that a patient could need, including a professional looking table tennis table.

My first day at The Friary was quiet, thankfully. When I arrived for duty in the afternoon the two female staff were making paper flowers for Christmas decorations. One of the nurses was a woman in her late fifties and she was soon to retire. She was an SEN. and very pleasant, though a bit ‘posh,’ I thought.

During the course of our first conversation I told her that I went to church, so thereafter Sally constantly referred to me as that good, clean living boy. I wasn’t a boy, though was I? I was a charge nurse, and was secretly rather irritated by this, especially as she continued in this vein right up until her retirement a few months later.

The other nurse was less pleasant and I never really liked her. She had a brittle northern accent. It transpired that her husband had disappeared some time earlier, and after seven years she had obtained a divorce, on the grounds that he could be dead. I felt sympathy towards her husband, if I had had the misfortune to be married to her, I would have disappeared too.

One day I happened to say to Sally that if I was left on the ward with just one nurse, which I frequently was, I would prefer it if it were a trained one. A day or so later I had only one nurse, Jessie, the sour face.

She was quiet for the early part of the shift, until at tea break I asked her if anything was wrong. She was like a ‘burning martyr,’ she seemed venomous and ‘hurt’ at the same time.

“I understand you don’t want me working with you,” she said coldly.

It took a lot of explaining to get her to see that I hadn't meant anything personal.

But I suppose that in my heart I did mean just that, as I found her quite unpleasant.

Because it was coming up to Christmas the ward was quiet and remained so for a couple of weeks, with no consultants rounds, only the odd one breezing in occasionally to see their private patients. I wasn't really sure what my role was at that time, so I was in the office a lot reading through the patients notes and trying to familiarise myself with the paperwork.

I surfaced at tea breaks of course, which were taken in the clinic room, a large room in the centre of the ward and the place where any of the patients went if they needed anything. That's where the other nurses usually were to be found, although I discovered early on that they were few and far between, we were severely understaffed. Usually I had Sally and Jessie, but it did often change on a daily basis, in fact anyone at all could turn up, which I didn't really feel was good for the patients, I felt that continuity of staff was better for them.

The nursing officer Mr. Mount was a pleasant man, even though a little effeminate. He always called me Brother Robert, unless I had upset him in some way, then it would be 'Mr. Panton.'

Mr. Mount was someone who in all the time I worked for him I couldn't really form any sort of relationship with at all. Highly strung and often touchy, he was in fact a man who wouldn't stand up for his nurses.

There were three acute admission wards in the hospital each having around twenty eight beds, but only two or three nurses on duty on any shift, with Mr. Mount responsible for doing the rota's.

There wasn't enough staff and I often told him so after I had been there for a while, he didn't try and rectify the situation, even when several of the senior staff went to see him with the same complaint. We were so short staffed that the management, instead of properly addressing the situation placed alarm bells on each ward, so that if there was an emergency we could get assistance from elsewhere.

I often said that the patients who got better did so in spite of us and not because of us. Apart from that easy period when I first arrived on the ward, it was a very hectic life and I didn't have nearly enough time to spend with the patients as I wanted and could really have done with some extra staff.

After the Christmas and New Year break the ward became very busy and I was able to take control and use my authority with the older staff, because we had a big influx of patients. Up until then I had been new boy and I felt I needed tread carefully and not upset the staff that had been there so much longer than I had, and in fact had a great deal more experience.

I remember one embarrassing experience that makes me blush even as I write. It was to do with one of the long stay patients, Thomas. He was a cousin of a baron and as such was held in awe by some. A nice man of few words, he had apparently been very disturbed when he arrived on the ward many years ago and had somehow obtained a can of black paint with which he painted his bed. Now, Thomas was an old man with an acute skin problem.

Sally told me one day that he needed a saline bath. I didn't know where to get the salt from, so I thought of the saline sachets in the clinic room and put some of those into his bath water. No one said anything, but later I thought 'silly me,' I should have gone and got some salt from the kitchen, because the little amount had contributed to the bath was as nothing at all.

The room that Thomas had slept in on his arrival and where the painting incident had taken place, was supposed to have been haunted. Many years before a man had lifted one of the feet of his bed up and let it fall onto his throat, thereby committing suicide. It was said that no one ever got better if they were put into that room, and actually it seemed to be true, even while I was there.

Another incident that I was involved in was with a ninety year old man who was suffering from retention of urine.

"Give him a diuretic," Sally suggested.

This was a tablet given to someone to help him or her rid themselves of unwanted fluids, especially if they had swollen ankles. It was something that only a doctor could prescribe. I gave it anyway because I thought Sally knew better than me. As a result the patient not only passed urine, but he passed it in such large quantities that he collapsed. The consultant happened to come onto the ward as I deliberated on what to do next, thinking it was the end of the line for me, especially as Thomas was a private patient.

"Don't worry," Dr. Hartley said, (he was the doctor I'd got to know two or three years earlier.) "He's going to be all right."

He was; the next day he had fully recovered much to my relief. I confessed to the doctor what I'd done and he just smiled and said,

"Well done."

I couldn't believe my luck.

One of the SEN's I worked with was Martha, she was an Irish nurse in her fifties and would often spend her tea breaks rubbing the varicose veins on her legs, with rolled down stockings, her husband had gone off with another woman and then decided that he would rather have Martha. She wasn't having any of it though, but kept him dangling on a string so as to get a new car whenever she needed one, as well as other expensive necessities.

I used to call her the Bowel Queen, because if we had an elderly admission and they were confused, she would give the patient an enema and miraculously that patient would often recover and be ready to be discharged within a few days, as the enema got rid of a build up of toxins. She was marvelous and I was very fond of her.

Martha had been at the hospital many years and she told me of how one of the old ladies that she'd nursed years ago remembered the soldiers passing by in the street on the way to the train station and to the trenches in the First World War.

Edna, another SEN. who I often worked with was particularly useful because she liked looking after the clinic and giving medicines out, or doing things like dressing wounds. This released me to deal with the many doctor's rounds, or listen to any patient that might have a particular problem.

Typical of many of our admissions was the middle age woman whose husband had retired and they found it difficult to cope with each other now they were both at home all the time.

We also had a lot of business people admitted who were finding life stressful. One of these was Stuart; he was fifty something and had several shops in town, which had managers in to run them. When he was first admitted he was suffering from pressure of speech and drove everyone crazy with his incessant, rapid talking. After he eventually settled down he told me that each one of his managers had been stealing from him and he was, as a result, in very serious financial difficulties. Stuart lived in a grand house that I passed on my way to work and had always admired. After his discharge this had to be sold and his businesses closed over the next few months to pay off his debts. After a while he was readmitted, but this time he was seriously depressed. His wife and he had parted and he didn't see any future. He was discharged again a few weeks later, apparently much better. Soon after he drove his car up a quiet country lane and committed suicide, a tragedy indeed.

Linda was a middle-aged lady who had recently lost her husband. While she was a patient on the ward she seemed to be reasonably content to sit and talk with the other women, but then she was told by the consultant that she had to go home for weekend leave. She whispered to me as she left the office,

"I'm a very sick woman you know, Robert."

Reluctantly she went home, only to take an overdose of sleeping pills that killed her.

It wasn't always all like that though, there were many success stories, and lots of people went home and never returned, having their mental health problems resolved.

There were others however who were long standing patients and they never seemed to be any different however many times they came to us. Rita was a good example; she was in a marriage that had never been happy although she'd worked at it for many years. As a result of her mental state she suffered physical symptoms, or so it seemed; no amount of tests could prove, or disprove it. She would come into Dr. Hartley's ward round week after week and complain of stomach pains.

"It ruckles your guts, Doctor." She would repeat week after week.

Dr. Hartley was always sympathetic and would keep her in for a few weeks to give her some respite from her unhappy existence, but as soon as he had left the office he would give me a knowing smile and shrug his shoulders.

He seemed to have a knack of landing himself with this sort of patient.

Another would come in and say,

"Well, you see doctor, its my stomach, it churns, its doing it now even while I'm talking to you."

She'd get hold of his hand and place it on her stomach.

"Can you feel the churning doctor?" she asked hopefully. Doctor Hartley, always truthful, had to confess that he couldn't.

As like so many of his ladies she came back to us time and time again. The doctor didn't seem to mind though; I think he rather liked the hero worship he received from them. He was very kind to his patients and of course unlike the other consultants he didn't have a retinue of junior doctors with him, it was just him, me and the patient at his ward rounds; all very intimate.

One of his patients was a woman in her late forties. He had a lot of time for her, especially as in the nineteen sixties, he confessed that he had treated her with LSD, a popular treatment, he said at that time. This had led Jean to become rather detached and remote and she was with us for long periods of time, but never showed any signs of improvement.

She would spend hours standing alone in the hospital library, where Dr. Hartley always saw her alone. He felt guilty about her condition and always blamed himself for it but as he told me there wasn't anything he could do to rectify the situation.

Chapter 20.

One of the most difficult things I had to deal with was the admission procedure. Usually it was ok. but sometimes it was really sad, as with the time when I admitted a young woman who was suffering with depression because she had been involved in a car crash where her husband and two children had been killed. She was the only survivor and didn't know how to cope with the guilt of being alive. As she told me her story I had to excuse myself and I rushed out of the office and into the toilet as I felt I would cry my eyes out; not very professional I know, but it wasn't the first, or the last time. I found it difficult to deal with these situations and often couldn't get to sleep at night thinking about them.

There was another woman who began sobbing when her mother was told that she would have to go into a nursing home and mothers house would have to be sold to pay for the cost of her care. The daughter was absolutely devastated as she had been counting on her inheritance to help pay off her own mortgage. Sometimes life didn't seem fair!

Despite these things I began to love the hospital and my job and wouldn't have wanted to be anywhere else, the stress notwithstanding. Even Mr. Mount my nursing officer seemed to be an acceptable part of my life.

He even forgave me when I overslept once and turned up for my shift three hours late. He wasn't quite so forgiving when one day I received a visit from a man who invited me to choose some new bedroom furniture. I saw no problem and went through the catalogue with him and chose what I thought appropriate for my ward.

A few hours later Mr. Mount came bursting through the office door breathing fire.

"Well, thankyou very, very much indeed," he fumed. "I thought you would have had the courtesy to involve me in the decision as to which furniture should be in my hospital."

To be quite honest I didn't know what to say. It all seemed so petty, and whose ward was it anyway? We agreed to disagree on that occasion!

There was also the time several of the patients had various medicines discontinued at a ward round, I couldn't for the life of me at that moment remember how to spell discontinued, so in the daily report that had to be sent to the nursing office I wrote that the medication had been 'knocked off.' I quite rightly received a sarcastic phone call from Mr. Mount asking me,

"What exactly do you mean by the expression 'knocked off,' Mr. Panton?"

Note that he didn't address me as 'Brother Robert' on that particular occasion!

Unfortunately the next incident wasn't so easy to deal with as I was most definitely in the wrong. One evening, believing he had gone home there was a very tempting sponge pudding going begging and so I hid myself in a corner of the kitchen and was tucking into it when Mr. Mount stuck his head around the corner.

"Oh, hello Mr. Mount," I spluttered through my illicit pudding, "I thought you'd gone home."

"Evidently," came the cold disapproving reply.

I was on holiday the next day, but knew that he wouldn't let it rest. It absolutely spoiled my time away with the family, and sure enough on my return he was waiting like a vulture for its prey.

Thankfully I didn't get the sack, but I knew I'd blotted my copy book and I had to be really good for a long time afterwards to make it up to him. My salvation came a few months later when we had the biggest snowfall in living memory. Despite the ten-foot snow drifts I trudged through the narrow track the snowplough had made to get to work one morning. Some of the other staff hadn't been able to make it, and as I lived four miles away I was looked upon as something of a hero. We worked with a skeleton staff for a couple of days and Mr. Mount was kindness itself to me after that.

If I thought the sponge pudding incident might end my career, something far more tragic put my job on the line during my time at the priory.

One afternoon several people were admitted one after another. I wasn't able to do all the paperwork myself so the SEN. who I was on duty with did some of it for me. I knew that we had at least two depressive women admitted that day, but because one of them had been in before and the other seemed more in need of attention, that's where I directed my attention. The other lady seemed to be quite happy talking to some of the other patients. Later I was to discover that she was known as a smiling depressive and although she appeared to be reasonably content, was in fact deeply depressed. On doing my nursing notes for the day, because it had been so busy, with only two staff on duty I omitted to write in this persons notes. During the night she committed suicide by strangling herself with a pair of tights.

When I came on duty the next morning the coroner had been and the body was taken away shortly afterwards. There was no excuse I could give and I was in deep trouble. I wasn't suspended, but was warned by a senior nursing officer from St. Andrews that there would be an enquiry and that my position was in danger.

I attended the coroner's inquest and gave evidence, and then a few days later went to attend a disciplinary hearing. My only plea was the shortage of staff and the pressure of work. This to some extent was accepted and I got away with a final written warning that was to last for one year.

In all of this I was desperately sorry for the family, but wasn't allowed to approach them. Even though I had made a tragic mistake, I felt that it was in fact because there wasn't enough staff on the ward, yet even after this, things didn't change for around another two years when Mr. Mount was eventually relieved of his position and demoted to charge nurse. Then we got a new nursing officer and more staff, but it was too late as the hospital was about to be run down and closed.

Before Mr. Mount left us I had just one more run in with him. It concerned a consultant, Dr. Ahmed who sent mostly older people to us. There was nothing wrong with that in principle, except that they often remained on the ward for months at a time and they grew in number. The consultants were complaining that there weren't enough beds, but when I explained the reason to them they didn't do anything about it, except chew my head off because they couldn't admit their very lucrative private patients.

Dr. Ahmed was a nice man, the fact that he was bed blocking couldn't take away from him the fact that he was easy going and a pleasure to deal with. He used to sit in the consulting room smoking his pipe and if anyone asked him a question he appeared to be enjoying the aroma of the tobacco so much that he often didn't answer for what seemed several minutes. I once jokingly said to one of the junior doctors that he'd got 'that Condor feeling.' Dr. Ahmed just looked at me, smiled and told me not to be cheeky.

But for all his endearing ways one day I felt I'd had enough. The ward was in total gridlock, because many of his elderly patients weren't able to leave due to social problems, such as needing sheltered accommodation, which was then as now difficult to come by.

His secretary telephoned to say that he wanted to admit an eighty something old lady onto the ward.

I said "No!""

Dr. Ahmed himself telephoned back and said, "I'm the consultant and I'm going to admit her."

I replied, "I don't care if you're the Queen of England, that patient isn't going to be admitted to my ward!"

The phone went dead, but it wasn't long before Mr. Mount came into my office, red faced and very annoyed. He was adamant that I was going to admit; I was just as sure that I wouldn't. We had a heated exchange and I thought that I would certainly get the sack. Fortunately Dr. Hamza, another consultant came in to see one of his patients and when I told him of my stand he immediately came to my rescue. The day was saved and the patient wasn't admitted.

Dr. Hamza was the consultant I'd upset while I was a student nurse, when I refused to do his ward round until the patients had eaten their lunch. At first when he saw I was the new charge nurse at The Friary he was very cool towards me, but he never said a word about the incident.

After a while he and I got on really well. That is except that he was a very volatile man and if I upset him he would give me a dressing down. Once he did it in the dining room in front of all the patients.

"Mr. Panton," he shouted angrily, "I'll have you sacked!"

I can't remember what I'd done to upset him, but I knew it was serious, as he usually called me Robert. I didn't get the sack, of course and everything was back to normal the next day.

Dr. Hamza was different from the other consultants, when he arrived on the ward with several junior doctors following behind him, everything had to grind to a halt so he could be given full attention. He was an arrogant man who would belittle his juniors, but for some reason everyone liked him, even myself who was often the butt of his egotistical sense of humour.

I remember one day confessing that I didn't know some elementary term and he took great delight in leaning back in his chair, cigarette in one hand and a cup of coffee in the other and saying,

"That's why, Mr. Panton, I'm a consultant and you are just a nurse."

Naturally this met with a round of laughter from the junior doctors, because they weren't the ones, for a change being put down.

He wasn't always right though; he once treated a patient for depression when she had cancer. She kept on telling him that she was in a great deal of pain, but he believed it was psychosomatic. It wasn't until a few weeks after the lady had been admitted that he'd agree to various tests to see if it was a physical disorder, by then it was too late anyway and the patient died.

One of his patients suffered from various phobias, including a fear of heights and as a private patient it was in his interest to cure him. He asked me if, on my days off I would take him to the top of various church towers and blocks of flats to help him conquer his fears. As he offered to pay me well for the service, I agreed. Over the next couple of weeks I took William, a young man in his early twenties up the highest places I could find; in lifts, up stairs and downstairs, then back again. I even took him to an air show, as he was supposed to be afraid of crowds too. Quite honestly I never thought he had any problems, he sailed through it all. I was getting well paid, so I had no complaints. When he was eventually discharged he gave Dr. Hamza some money to give towards the ward funds as a 'Thankyou.' He obviously felt that he had benefited from his stay with us.

Dr. Hamza dealt with a number of private patients who had long-term drug abuse problems. I was quite used to giving injections and even taking blood in the absence of the phlebotomist, but when I was asked to give vitamin injections to several of his patients, I came across something that I'd never encountered before. Their buttocks were like cardboard. I could hardly get the needle in. I couldn't, and still don't understand why. I was under the impression that most people who injected drugs used their arms, but those people must have used their buttocks over and over again!

James, the GP. who knew his trees was a frequent admission to Shackleton, as was Michael a man who also had an alcohol problem and had been my boss when, as a teenager I worked briefly in a hardware shop. His was a very sad case. The family business that he had inherited on his father's death had been around for over a hundred and fifty years, but his parents had both drunk much of it away by the time Michael came into possession of it. It was a terrible tragedy that he too came to like the demon drink too much, so much so that the firm went bankrupt.

Michael was one of life's gentlemen and I thought a lot of him, despite the fact that I often found half empty bottles of whisky hidden in his room on each occasion he was a patient at the Friary. One night I was walking home from church and a car came suddenly to a halt at the side of me. Michael literally fell out laughing, much the worse for drink. I helped him up to his flat and was invited inside. it was so sad to see so little left, as I had been to his childhood home and had seen all the antiques and expensive furniture. The only thing that was of any value now was the grandfather clock.

Michael died a little while after. I'm sure his that children and the wife who had divorced him years before because, she couldn't take any more, must have mourned him.

Chapter 21.

After five and a half years of working at The Friary I had the opportunity of taking a part time position as a minister in a local evangelical church and after much deliberation I took the post. It meant going onto night duty as a staff nurse which I negotiated with my new nursing officer.

What a release it was, I hadn't realised the pressure I'd been under and now felt that I was a new person. The last few years had been hard, with taking on the problems of the patients and working understaffed for much of the time. I still had the responsibility, but to a much lesser degree. Mostly the patients were in bed by midnight and apart from the odd one who needed someone to talk to at night it was much easier going.

The nurse in charge of the hospital on night duty became a good friend and because the hospital was nearing the end of its life the archaeologists were invited into the grounds to do some research. The Friary was situated close to where the Romans had settled centuries before and its site was of special historic interest. Alfie was keen on using a metal detector, so he would bring his own state of the art machine and another, rather inferior thing for me to use and we'd spend our breaks, torch in hand looking for hoards of roman coins. We never found any of course, but it was exciting.

The archaeologists had dug a number of trenches and came across a medieval burial ground. We would lift up the plastic sheets they'd placed in the trenches, and often we'd find a skull grinning up at us. We spent hours with the detectors scanning the ground where the work was being done, but only found a large brass buckle and something that looked like it may have come off a roman centurions helmet.

Another of Alfie's interest was photography and we would spend a lot of time taking long exposure pictures of paintings and furniture that were in abundance throughout the hospital.

We still had the patients to look after of course, but they could sometimes seem like an intrusion into our nocturnal activities, especially if they were noisy and disruptive, as some of them were on occasions, it could be a problem at night when staffing levels were low.

One girl in particular used to set the fire alarms off during the early hours, causing mayhem, as the fire service was obliged to attend with blue lights flashing, much to the annoyance of the local residents, some of whom complained and after several nights of this she had to be locked in her room during the night for a week or two, so everyone could have some peace.

Another young woman who was suffering from hypo mania and couldn't sleep had to have a nurse assigned to her for a number of nights otherwise she would run through the dormitories waking all the other patients up.

Still it was a much calmer life for me, but it wasn't to last. After around a year we were called to a meeting and told that the hospital was to close. We knew it was coming, but what a miserable time it was for those who'd spent most of their working lives there. Not to mention the distress to the patients, especially the long term ones. The process didn't take long, and after a few short weeks, while I was away on holiday the front door closed on over one hundred and sixty years of history. The hospital was empty and silent for the first time in all those years.

Minnie was sent up to St. Andrews where I saw her after a while, she was truly miserable as she thought that the other patients were vulgar and she wouldn't have anything to do with them if she could help it.

Thomas was given a place in a nursing home and died within three days.

Martha another patient who'd been on Shackleton for many years was transferred to a nursing home too, where all the money she had inherited from her fathers estate was swallowed up in care costs. She lived for three or four years, but wasn't happy by all accounts.

I was particularly unhappy about Martha, because she was so harmless and endearing. If she were asked how she was she would always reply,

"I'm a lot better now. Thank you nurse."

To me it seemed tragic that someone who'd been there for so many years and was loved by not only the staff, but by the other patients, who were like her family, should end up the way she did.

Most of the other patients went home as the hospital was run down; some were sent to the same ward as Minnie, the rest dispersed throughout the hospital wherever there was a suitable place.

I was to work at St. Andrews until it also closed just like The Friary; At first I didn't like it as I had become used to the much more comfortable surroundings of The Friary since working at St. Andrews as a student. Eventually, though it became like home to me again. I had a friend on night duty who would bring his guitar along and we would find some quiet corner in our breaks and have a singsong. A lot of the staff came from The Friary, but many took early retirement, or found other jobs, because it was so different that they never felt as if they belonged at St. Andrews.

After The Friary had been shut down for sometime and before it was turned into a museum I was asked to go to collect something that had been left behind.

Turning the key in the lock I knew I wouldn't like what I was to see inside. It was a cold day outside and colder in the reception area. I put the article I'd retrieved to one side and climbed the stairs to Shackleton as I had done so many times before, remembering the day I'd slipped whilst on my way down and twisted my ankle because I was so eager to collect my pay slip.

It was deathly quiet and I could almost hear the ghostly voices of the past century and a half calling out in protest as I walked slowly along the corridor towards my old office. Under my feet the carpet crunched with all the dirt that had accumulated over the months. I looked at the space where Minnie had sat, now it was bare and sad. She had been so full of opinions on classical music and the arts. She had a delusion that she was called to bring peace to the world and often asked me what I thought of George Orwell and his 'Big Brother' theory. Now all of her thoughts and opinions were a miserable memory.

I recalled how I had tried to get her out of bed in the mornings.

"In just a moment," she would murmur sleepily, over and over again, as I made repeated trips to her room, often six or seven times in the morning; she'd be up by eleven o clock if I were lucky.

Then there was old Thomas' place. He had been so settled at The Friary; now he was dead, probably because he had had to move on to a place that was so unlike that which he had been used to.

I found myself in the office, so empty now and so dirty. It had never been dirty, I spent many hours over the years just dusting and cleaning the windows so I could get a better view of the old church in the distance. What stories that old office could tell. Way before my time there would be people pouring out their troubles to the nurses and the doctors, now it was just a silent, sad memory.

I closed the front door of the hospital after I'd finished and trudged back to my car recalling the days that were gone now. In those days I'd walk around the surrounding streets in my lunch breaks just for the sheer joy of soaking up all the history of the area.

St. Andrews was to go the same way. Within a couple of years all the patients had been re-homed in little units in, or around the town. Some would go into nursing homes, or maybe into houses in the community, the acute patients by now had their own unit attached to the general hospital.

Others committed suicide rather than leave. One man climbed the water tower that stood close by the main building and threw himself off, another found an old air raid shelter nearby and hung himself. I don't know of any female patients who did similar things, but I wouldn't be surprised if there were some. Quite a few patients would rather die than leave the place that had, in some cases been their home and their family and their sense of belonging and acceptance for many years.

St. Andrews, where my great grandfather had worked was emptied and then for the greater part demolished. I know that there were a lot of bad things about the place, but there was an awful lot of good; now though, for better, or worse it is consigned to history. That is, apart from the memories it has for myself and for many others who were there as staff, or as patients. That's why I wanted to write about it, just so that those who might read this can get a flavour of how it was, and also so that St. Andrews, The Friary and all the other mental hospitals that have been closed down over these past twenty years, or so aren't forgotten.

Memory is a funny thing and even though there were a lot of things that weren't right in the old hospitals I, like many of those patients and staff thought that there was an atmosphere that couldn't be replicated elsewhere, and it was a sad day to see it all pass away.